Medical and Biological Engineering in the Future of Health Care

•

Edited by J.D. Andrade

University of Utah Press
Salt Lake City, Utah

LIBRARY OF CONGRESS CATALOGING-IN-PUBLICATION DATA

Medical and biological engineering in the future of health care /
edited by Joseph D. Andrade.
p.   cm.
Includes bibliographical references and index.
ISBN 0-87480-454-X (acid-free paper)
1. Biomedical engineering. I. Andrade, Joseph D., 1941–   .
R856.M36   1994
610'.28—dc20   94-8413

Contents

Foreword

The roles of bioengineering and of medical technologies in the health care system are certainly not new topics. Some of the topics addressed in this volume have been discussed in other forums at other times, but all too often with limited audiences and with no permanent record or follow-up of the discussions. However, recently the escalating cost of health care has catapulted technology to center stage. Everywhere one travels in this country, one finds the general public very concerned about their own personal health care problems and confused about the contribution of technology to health care.

The American Institute for Medical and Biological Engineering (AIMBE) was formed several years ago to provide a unified and coherent representation of the field and to deal with problems that are important to all areas of medical and biological engineering and our affiliated societies. A major purpose of AIMBE is to establish the scholarly and professional identity of medical and biological engineering and to speak for this discipline on issues of concern to the American people. In 1993 the delivery of health care—technology, economics, and management—dominated the political agenda. Therefore, AIMBE's second annual event, held at the National Academy of Sciences on March 8–9, 1993, was devoted to "The Future of Health: The Role of Medical and Biological Engineering."

It is AIMBE's intent to promote the engineering approach to medicine and to involve medical and biological engineers in addressing health and well-being through the development and appropriate use of technology. As part of its mission, AIMBE hopes to act as a catalyst in involving the community; to conduct research on issues related to the evaluation, development, and appropriate use of technology; to formulate recommendations on public policy; and to educate professionals as well as the public at large.

In the United States, the interface of engineering with medicine is quite effective at the research level. It is also demonstrably successful from the viewpoint of product development, as evidenced by American dominance of the biotechnological and medical-product industries. The interface is much weaker at the level of clinical application and clinical evaluation of medical technology. Engineering, biology, and medicine have not yet come together to address the new societal concern for technology assessment.

To much of the public, the uncontrolled use of health care technology seems directly linked to the escalation of health care costs. Some health care professionals and national policymakers implicate engineering developments as a root cause of the problem. They fail to see how, in the proper framework, the use of technology can improve health and quality of life at an affordable cost. To most, the contribution of biomedical engineering to that worthy goal is not apparent.

This volume is intended as a first step in AIMBE's effort to document the contribution of engineering to human and environmental health. Its objective will be achieved if the reader comes to appreciate the place of medical technology in health care and to identify some of the factors—economic, demographic, and cultural—which condition the appropriate utilization of medical technologies.

Pierre Galletti
President-elect, AIMBE
and
Robert Nerem
President, AIMBE

Preface

JOSEPH ANDRADE
University of Utah

"The fact that man is mortal ... is not well appreciated in our society."

"Everything in our society that goes haywire or is negative is someone else's responsibility."

"There has been little or no attention given to the cost implications ... of new medical technologies. ... Those days are now clearly over."

"[M]otivate, mobilize, and otherwise encourage the medical and biological engineering community to seriously look at its collective and its individual objectives and actions in light of current national needs and concerns."

The health care debate currently rages. Access to health care, the quality of health care, and particularly the costs of health care in the United States were major issues in the last presidential election and are major priorities in the Clinton administration. Concern for the costs and quality of health care is not limited to the United States. It is an international concern for every major nation in the world faced with the problem of escalating health care costs.

Although the figures depend on what you read, who you listen to, and the numbers you believe, almost all believe that a major component of the overall costs of health care in this country is administrative bureaucracy and inefficiency, due in part to the several thousand individual and somewhat independent insurance companies and the excessive paperwork that plagues all parts of society—providers and patients alike.

Other major components of the costs of care are due to the litigiousness of society in the United States and to the practice of defensive medicine. The fact that the U.S. has more lawyers per capita than any other nation, and that these lawyers are accustomed to or expectant of a well-to-do life-style and quality of life, increases the level of litigation and complicates an already complex problem.

Another factor is that the general population, including lawyers and physicians, basically has a very poor understanding of health benefits versus risks. The fact that man is mortal—that concerns of life, health, disease, and others are managed in large part by statistics—is not well appreciated in our society.

Also, as related in two recent editorials in *Newsweek*,[1] it seems that everything in our society that goes haywire or is negative is often viewed as someone else's responsibility. If I smoke and get lung cancer, it is the cigarette industry's responsibility. If I slip on the ice in a shopping mall parking lot, it is that shopping mall's responsibility. If my child watches too much television, particularly too much TV violence, it is the TV network's responsibility; and, of course, if my operation takes a bad turn, it is the physician's and the hospital's responsibility, and I have a right to sue—and I expect to get a substantial award. Statistics don't matter in the case of my personal problems. Things are seen as either black or white. It, of course, cannot be my responsibility; so it must be yours.

These are the general issues and problems which are at the heart of our health care crisis, and are also at the heart of many of our other societal problems.

Health policy, health economics, and technology assessment professionals often say that increased application of technologies is responsible for a major part of escalating health care costs. It is important to understand that in health care policy circles, medical technologies are practically everything not included in the eighteenth-century physician's black bag. The concept includes any and all chemical diagnostics, all physical diagnostic instruments, all drugs and pharmaceuticals, and all medical devices.

Modern medical technologies are generally developed by

universities, research hospitals, and industrial research and development (R&D) laboratories. These technologies are further developed, engineered, and tested by industries, and are then aggressively sold and marketed to health care providers. Those responsible for the ideas, inception, and the early development of such technologies are generally physicians, biomedical engineers, and/or industrial research scientists and engineers.

Although undergraduate engineering programs do indeed consider the economics and cost-benefit aspects of engineering activities and products, such considerations are not generally included in medical school or graduate engineering programs. It is safe to say that in the great majority of graduate biomedical engineering programs in the United States there has been little or no attention given to the cost implications—particularly the overall health care cost implications—of the development, diffusion, and application of new medical technologies. The same can be said for medical schools' programs. However, those days are now clearly over.

The academic, clinical medicine, and industrial research and development communities are now well aware that there is a health care cost problem. We are all in part responsible for it, although we often console ourselves by suggesting that lawyers and insurance companies are responsible for far more of it. Yet we as professionals have a responsibility to change the way we practice bioengineering and the way we practice medicine.

The conference from which this book was derived was the outgrowth of a recommendation made by an NSF-Whitaker Foundation workshop, held in April 1992 and organized by Dov Jaron and Peter Katona.[2]

The conference had substantial discussion after each major talk, as well as several extensive panel discussions. In this volume some of the panelist statements have been incorporated in edited form as short papers. The remainder of the panel discussion and the individual discussions after each major talk have been very briefly summarized by the editor and included after the appropriate chapter.

The major objective of the meeting was to provide perspective and background for AIMBE's members and guests. Speakers were chosen who, in addition to providing comprehensive and authoritative overviews and perspectives, would also motivate, mobilize, and otherwise encourage the medical and biological engineering community to seriously look at its collective and its individual objectives and actions in light of current national needs and concerns. We think this book meets those objectives.

AIMBE's Board of Directors and the Conference Program Committee (Gilbert Devey, Richard Johns, Jerome Schultz, Clifford Goodman, Kenneth Keller, Robert Nerem, and Louis Sheppard) join me in acknowledging the involvement and participation of the other discussants, introducers, and session chairs: Joseph Bordogna, Donald Detmer, Pierre Galletti, Edward Hinman, Peter Katona, Winfred Phillips, Lawrence Shearon, and John Watson.

Financial support was provided by the Whitaker Foundation, the National Science Foundation, the Hugoton Foundation, and the American Institute for Medical and Biological Engineering. Pfizer and Becton Dickinson also provided financial assistance. We also thank the National Academy of Sciences leadership and staff for their excellent help.

Completion of this volume was aided immeasurably by Stephen Kern of the University of Utah, who videotaped the entire meeting. Lisa Marley Baker did most of the transcription; Cindi Dunford and Mindy Steadman prepared the final manuscript, and the staff of the University of Utah Press produced the book. We also thank Dr. Louis Sheppard and Debbie Gohmert of the University of Texas, Galveston, and Michael Murphy in R. Nerem's office at Georgia Tech for the local arrangements and successful conducting of the conference.

References

1. R.J. Samuelson, "The Excuse Industry," *Newsweek* (December 11, 1989): 74; and M. Greenfield, "Playing the Blame Game," *Newsweek* (May 28, 1990): 82.

2. J.D. Andrade, D. Jaron, and P. Katona, "Improved Delivery and Reduced Costs of Health Care Through Engineering," *IEEE Engineering in Medicine and Biology* (June, 1993): 38–41.

ABBREVIATIONS

AAAS:	American Association for the Advancement of Science
ACR-NEMA:	American College of Radiology—North America Equipment Manufacturer's Association
AHCPR:	Agency for Health Care Policy and Research
AICHE:	American Institute of Chemical Engineers
AIMBE:	American Institute for Medical and Biological Engineering
AMA:	American Medical Association
AMIA:	American Medical Informatics Association
ANSI:	American National Standards Institute
ARPA:	Advanced Research Projects Agency
ASAIO:	American Society for Artificial Internal Organs
ASTM:	American Society for Testing and Materials
ATP:	Adenosine Triphosphate
BMES:	Biomedical Engineering Society
BOD:	Biological Oxygen Demand
BPH:	Benign Prostatic Hyperplasia
CAT:	Computer-aided Tomography
CBER:	Center for Biologics Evaluation Research
CCD:	Charge Coupled Device
CD:	Circular (Optical) Disc
CDER:	Center for Drug Evaluation Research
CHOLE:	Cholecystectomy
CPI:	Clinical Practice Improvement
CPR:	Computer-Based Patient Record
CPRI:	Computer-Based Patient Record Institute
CQI:	Continuous Quality Improvement
CT:	Computer Tomography
DICOM:	Digital Imaging and Communications in Medicine
DOE:	Department of Energy
DRG:	Diagnosis Related Groups
DSA:	Digital Subtraction Angiography
EC:	European Community
ECG:	Electrocardiograms
EMG:	Electromyogram
EPA:	Environmental Protection Agency

ER:	Emergency Room
FDA:	Food and Drug Administration
FET:	Field Effect Transistor
GDP:	Gross Domestic Product
GI:	Gastrointestinal
GME:	General Medical Expenses
GNP:	Gross National Product
HCTI:	Health Care Technology Institute
HIMA:	Health Industry Manufacturers Association
HIPC:	Health Insurance Purchasing Cooperatives
HMO:	Health Maintenance Organization
HPCC:	High Performance Computing and Communication
IC:	Integrated Circuit
ICMIT:	International Consortium for Medical Imaging Technology
IEEE:	Institute of Electronic and Electrical Engineers
IHC:	Intermountain Health Care (Salt Lake City)
IITA:	Information Infrastructure Applications and Technology
IND:	Investigational New Drug
IOM:	Institute of Medicine
IRB:	Institutional Review Board
ISO:	International Standards Organization
LAN:	Local Area Network
LAP:	Laparoscopy
MIDAS:	Medical Information Display and Analyses System
MIT:	Massachusetts Institute of Technology
MR:	Magnetic Resonance
NAS:	National Academy of Sciences
NASA:	National Aeronautics and Space Administration
NEMA:	North American Equipment Manufacturers Association
NIH:	National Institutes of Health
NIST:	National Institute of Standards and Technology
NLM:	National Library of Medicine
NOAA:	National Oceanics and Atmospheric Administration
NREN:	National Research and Education Network
NSF:	National Science Foundation
OR:	Operating Room
OSHA:	Occupational Safety and Health Administration
OSTP:	Office of Science and Technology Policy
OTA:	Office of Technology Assessment
PACS:	Picture Archival and Communications Systems
PC:	Personal Computer
PET:	Positron Emission Tomography

PORT:	Patient Outcomes Research Team
QALY:	Quality Adjusted Life Years
RFP:	Request for Proposal
RIS:	Radiology Information System
ROM:	Read Only Memory
RMR:	Regenstriel Medical Record
RSNA:	Rehabilitation Society of North America
SAW:	Surface Acoustic Wave
SPECT:	Single Photon Emission Computer Tomography
TUIP:	Transurethral Incisional Prostatectomy
TURP:	Transurethral Prostatectomy
UK:	United Kingdom
VA:	Veterans Administration
WAN:	Wide Area Network

PART I

·

PERSPECTIVES ON MEDICAL TECHNOLOGY AND HEALTH CARE

CHAPTER 1

Prioritizing Biomedical Technologies

SAMUEL THIER
Brandeis University

"What the system should be doing is providing the proper balance of screening, prevention, diagnosis, treatment, and rehabilitation."

"Technology is neither cost-enhancing nor cost-saving. Certain technologies increase costs, certain technologies reduce costs."

"There is almost nothing I did as an intern and resident that is still the standard practice. The reason is that biomedical technology has made it possible to do more things more effectively and more safely than ever before—but at a cost."

"We have a calculus which confines us to a separation of the ledger. We don't make decisions which are in the best interest of the public. . . . We do not do proper assessment of the costs avoided; and the costs avoided are not simply within the medical system but within society as a whole. Since health costs are spread over the entire society, the health benefits should be spread and analyzed in the same way."

What is a high-priority biomedical technology? It should:
- be truly new;
- address prevention or cure of a problem;
- correct a great disease burden;
- improve net health outcome by having an enormous effect on each individual patient or person;
- be the obvious choice from among many for the particular circumstance;
- substitute for all previous choices;
- be easy to perform;
- have minimal invasive qualities and minimal side effects or risks; and
- be very inexpensive compared to what it replaces.

If you have that technology, go right ahead and use it! The problem, however, is that life is just not that simple.

The perspective presented here might be somewhat different from the perspective derived from an engineering basis. We will compare the engineering perspective and the medical perspective, because we need an equilibrium between the two if we want to determine priorities and move forward.

The broadest definition of medical technology includes:
- medical devices and instrumentation,
- pharmaceuticals and biologicals,
- diagnostic and therapeutic procedures,
- care systems, and
- information management systems.

These are all part of the technology of medicine and they are all included in this overview, although they may not be susceptible to the same prioritization or the same kinds of analyses.

Why is this a matter of concern to engineers, health professionals, economists, public policy experts, and the public in general? We are, for the first time in several decades (but not for the first time in our history), engaging the health care system and seeing whether we can reform a system which we take to be out of control. The reasons we identify it as being out of control are that:
- there are limits to access;
- we have what many consider to be an unacceptable set of public-health statistics, including life expectancy and infant mortality; and
- the costs are higher than those of any other nation.

Medical technology is frequently blamed as one of the key cost culprits.

Those who are involved in the generation and use of technology are nervous and concerned that health care reform may decrease our capacity to continue to develop, introduce, and use biomedical technologies. It is fascinating to me that technology is seen as a prime culprit in this arena, because it was not very long ago that it was seen as the promise for the future. It is now viewed by many as too expensive and, even when it is beneficial, overused.

As a physician, I learned that new technologies often would come at us too fast, before they were adequately evaluated and/or faster than we could assimilate them into our own framework of use. The physician would tend to use the additional technology until s/he learned whether it really was an adequate replacement for the old. During that period of disequilibrium a physician would likely be using multiple technologies in order to obtain a result that one of the technologies, if properly understood, alone would have provided. The data was not available which would give you the assurance that a new technology was the best one to use, so your comfort in using it in your practice was also missing. The pace at which technology can be assimilated becomes important. Technology has been oversold and underregulated (at least in regard to safety and efficacy). This is not stated as truth but as criticism and reflects reasons why people are worried about technology.

The range of criticism suggests that there must be some truth to some of them. An editorial I wrote several years ago about manpower policy in health was titled "Base it on facts, not opinions."[1] The same plea should be made for medical technology. There are many opinions and selective data analyses which profess to show one thing or another about technology and its impact on medical costs. The sets of questions are rarely adequately framed, however, and the analysis therefore is frequently misleading.

I graduated from medical school in 1960. Since that time, preventive services have improved dramatically. The statistical and epidemiologic underpinnings for preventive activities are dramatically better today than they were thirty years ago. We are developing more and better vaccines, and we have improved our capacity to screen, in terms of the overall number of conditions for which we can screen and the accuracy of the screening. We have developed new tests which can be diagnostic and monitor the care provided.

They are automated, reducing the unit costs, and they are more accurate. The area of imaging has been completely revolutionized with CT scanning, MRIs, and PET scans. Fiber optics have been added and widely disseminated. There are new pharmaceuticals and whole new classes of drugs for cardiovascular disease. There are new groups of antibiotics as well as new groups of chemotherapeutic and immunosuppressive agents. Transplantation surgery developed broadly—artificial organs, rehabilitation, and information management has become a critical part of what we do. There is almost nothing I did as an intern and resident that is still the standard practice. The reason is that biomedical technology has made it possible to do more things, more effectively, and more safely than ever before—but at a cost.

What is the cost? Before we try to answer that question we must consider a few cultural biases. First is the resistance to technology. "It will never come into general use and its value is extremely doubtful, because its beneficial application requires much time and gives a good bit of trouble to both the patient and practitioner and because its human character are foreign and opposed to all our habits and associations." That is a quotation from an 1834 editorial in the *London Times* about the introduction of the stethoscope! The public's resistance to technology is high and has always been so. Other kinds of biases creep in as well.

One of my favorite colleagues, Lewis Thomas, wrote a wonderful essay on technology[2] in which he describes *supportive technology* as that which produces comfort. He defines *halfway technologies*, in which he includes dialysis and pacemakers; and he defines *high technology*, which includes the replacement of a missing hormone or a vaccination. He maintains the enormous expenses of halfway technology have to be converted into basic research in order that the full technology of prevention or complete cure is possible. Squandering monies on halfway technology is not the proper policy, he argues. His views generated a tremendous amount of attention. He then wrote another essay entitled "My Magical Metronome,"[3] which many people have not read and which I never hear quoted. He describes developing a fluttering feeling in his chest, going into the hospital, and finding himself to be in complete heart block. He is put on a cardiac monitor in a coronary care unit, and, in classic Lew Thomas style, he writes that he looked up at the monitor and thought "The handwriting on the wall. And illiterate at that." He then describes having the pacemaker put in and his enormous pride at watching the pacemaker blip and his heart respond in time. He is proud of himself for following this magic metronome, and he recants; he says that halfway technology, when you need it, is very, very useful. What we need is a balance between the two—between halfway technology with its enormous expense and noncorrective function, but with the capacity to move people back to functional, autonomous lives, and high technology that moves us ahead towards prevention and cure.

There are a few issues facing us if we want to analyze where we are going in our efforts at prioritizing biomedical technology. The benchmarks we must consider are safety and efficacy or effectiveness. Efficacy is what happens in controlled circumstances; effectiveness is what happens when the technology gets out into general use. If you have a lethal illness, then safety is a different kind of choice than if we are considering a technology that adds a minor increment to that which is already present, technology that is a little more expensive and a little more risky.

The capacity for choice, particularly patient choice, becomes critical and must not be lost. Cost is important, particularly incremental cost. We must look at what we are getting for the additional cost relative to what we already have and the benefits provided.

We must ask whether the problems we have with technology are intrinsic to the technology, or are intrinsic to its use. The technology may have, as part of its use, a certain set of risks, complications, or breakdowns. We also must consider the application of the technology in practice. It is very dangerous to penalize the technology if the issue is regulation or application. It would be a shame to forego a useful technology when the focus should instead be on improving the way it is used, disseminated, or regulated.

Let me approach this problem as a physician by looking primarily at clinical need. What is it we are trying to accomplish? In the final analysis, we are looking at the maintenance or return of health as the goal of biomedical technology.

Consider screening, prevention, diagnosis, treatment, and rehabilitation. Screening is the kind of thing you can do with testing for HIV, by looking for antibodies in the blood supply, or by looking at populations of individuals. Mammography is another form of screening. Both are extremely effective and each has major policy debates associated with it: with HIV it is the intrusion of personal privacy; with mammography it is the growing debate about whether it really is worthwhile and effective. For those at age fifty and above there does not seem to be much debate, but there is considerable debate as to the advisability of such screening for women in their forties. These are the kinds of questions where data will help. Then the technology can be appropriately applied. One must not overuse the technology if the data show that it should not be used. In prevention we have enormous amounts of information now about smoking, diet, exercise, but we have little data on behavioral modification and the capacity to translate that knowledge into real usefulness for the population. Nevertheless, the smoking incidence among adults in this country has dropped below that of most other countries. Diagnosis, using imaging, is probably the best example of how we have converted from invasive to non-invasive technology and enhanced our accuracy at the same time. Conceptualize that spectrum of activities. Now place different engineered approaches into those different categories. We will invest more in priorities in one of those areas than another in relation to what we wish to accomplish.

How do we evaluate the technology? There are two levels of analysis. One is the controlled clinical trial, used typically by the pharmaceutical industry. The other is post-diffusion assessment, which is critical. Some devices get modified in use, and the skills of those using them become important parts of the evaluation. Further diffusion should then be dependent on the evaluation. Since we cannot evaluate everything developed by technology, we must determine characteristics of the technology that would make it most useful to be evaluated:

- Does it improve the outcome of a patient's treatment?
- Could it be applied to large patient populations?
- Does it address an important disease burden?
- Does it attempt to reduce risk?
- Does it reduce variation in practice?
- Does it reduce unit or aggregate costs?

To the extent that it meets these criteria, a new technology would be selected for evaluation, and one would couple the evaluation to the approval—the simplest approval being that of reimbursement. The reimbursement structure will, to a great extent, control the diffusion of technology. But it is important not to delay diffusion, as we did for CT scanning, which has been well demonstrated to be a great benefit to the public. It is also important not to move things through too quickly. If we are going to do the evaluation and get to the issue of costs, I believe we should use a broader calculus than we have been using heretofore.

Technology is neither necessarily cost-enhancing nor cost-saving. Certain technologies increase costs, certain technologies reduce costs. Unless you examine the individual technologies you can't answer the question. A classic example is prenatal care. There is very good evidence that adequate prenatal care preventing low birth weight will prevent or reduce the use of very intensive neonatal special care—that for every dollar invested you might save three dollars. The problem is that the person investing one dollar is not the person saving three dollars. The people who could have invested one dollar did not because we have a calculus that confines us to a separation of the ledger. We often don't make decisions which are in the best interest of the public.

A simple example is the lithotripter. This shock-wave disrupter of stones, most effective for kidney stones, is an expensive machine to put in place. Per treatment cost may be relatively significant—certainly the up-front costs are significant—but, if you were to get the patient out of the hospital in 24 to 48 hours, as opposed to a week or ten days, the cost to the health care system is rather impressively reduced. If, in addition, you get the person back to work in one week versus four weeks, then the change in productivity and time lost from work becomes an important component in the calculus. A more comprehensive economic impact needs to be built into the cost-benefit assessment.

We have developed the view that if something is expensive then that cost is *added*. We do not do a proper assessment of the costs avoided; and the costs avoided are not simply within the medical system but within society as a whole. Since health costs are spread over the entire society, the health benefits should be spread and analyzed in the same way. That is not now the case. In addition, the "cost" benefits in relief of pain, reassurance, decrease of anxiety, and general patient satisfaction are a set of parameters which need to be somehow quantified or at least considered and made part of the calculus of the evaluation of a new technology.

Why bother? Because we face enormous technologic promise —a biologic revolution. My friends in the engineering and physical sciences don't like me to say it, but biological sciences are now at the end of this century what physics was at the beginning of the century. It is *the* exciting science, the open frontier, the place to which some of the brightest young people are being attracted. What that might mean is beyond our imagination.

Could any of us have imagined in 1960 where we now stand today? It would be silly to predict what kinds of things are going to be happening in thirty years. But it is not hard to see the general directions. Consider the genome project. By 1995 we hope to have all the genes mapped, and in the next many years we will have their sequences. We will then know the proteins which are genetic predisposing factors for illness and resistance; we will develop the capacity to measure those markers and predict susceptibility and resistance to disease at a level we cannot imagine today. Think of what that might mean in terms of potential screening programs and in preventive services. We will also be able to improve our ability to diagnose, treat, and track diseases. We will be able to identify and replace missing proteins. We may replace them at first by making new biologics and getting them into patients. It is almost certain that later we will engineer the cells that patients will need to maintain the production of those proteins. Thus a whole series of illnesses can be corrected. These things are not beyond the realm of imagination at this point. We are moving in that direction.

Bioengineering will extend beyond what we are talking about in medicine into the nutritional area. The capacity to bioengineer foods will have enormous impact, both in this country and in developing countries. Behavioral science will be reinvigorated. We may be able to teach people to change their behaviors in their own defense. We will look for continued reductions in invasiveness and improvements in imaging techniques. We will have better-engineered devices.

We likely will see some further constrictions on the regulation of devices. Although public opinion is driving such constriction, there still will be continued improvements and expansion of devices. Devices will be of enormous help in the field of rehabilitation. The new molecular biology will allow us to begin to look at nerve regeneration and the correction of neurologic injury.

We will require the capacity to manage vast sums of information; the computer sciences will become progressively more important, both in information management and also in the capacity to manage the systems of care which will need to be integrated if we are really going to have health system reform.

Our approach to health system reform is again making the same mistake that we have made *every* time, which is to say "We will define the global budget and thus control costs," without asking what the system should be doing.

What the system should be doing is providing the proper balance of screening, prevention, diagnosis, treatment, and rehabilitation. When it begins to ask questions about the proper balance, then the technologies that relate to those various components of the system will be the technologies that you will prioritize.

References

1. S.O. Thier and R.W. Berliner, "Manpower Policy: Base It on Facts, Not Opinions," *New England Journal of Medicine*, 299:1305–7.

2. L. Thomas, *The Lives of a Cell* (New York: Bantam Books, 1974), 35–42.

3. L. Thomas, *Late Night Thoughts on Listening to Mahler's Ninth Symphony* (New York: Bantam Books, 1984), 45–48.

4. K.B. Ekelman, ed., *New Medical Devices* (Washington, D.C.: National Academy Press, 1988).

•

CHAPTER 2

•

Issues in the Development and Adoption of Technology in Medicine

KENNETH H. KELLER
Council on Foreign Relations

"Our strategy was one of 'technology push' rather than 'societal pull'—what we developed and marketed was whatever engineering ingenuity could create."

"How people perceive risk, and how they approach its management, is very much a function of how they view technology.... To the extent that society is alienated from technology, it will hold it to a much higher standard with respect to risk.... No technology is risk free."

"Society's view of liability is quite different with respect to a machine than it is with respect to a human being.... Society insists upon reductions in risk potential to unrealistically low levels.... Can the biomedical engineering community help to promote societal acceptance of a more realistic approach to risk?"

"The litigiousness of our society leads to what is sometimes called 'defensive medical practices,' erring on the side of more rather than less."

"The cost of a given technology always decreases and its effectiveness increases over time. . . . Cost-effectiveness comparisons made at the time of introduction of a technology will always be misleading. If adverse decisions are made on the basis of that initial comparison, the ultimate benefit will be lost."

"Data bases may have the greatest potential for reducing medical costs of any single kind of technology."

"Cost-effectiveness as a concept has some serious limitations in terms of the values of the society."

"What is needed is the social equivalent of an environmental impact statement."

The past, it has been remarked, is often no more than prologue. The 1989 meeting of the American Society for Artificial Internal Organs is a case in point.[1] At a symposium on the first morning of that conference, a number of people who frequently spoke at those meetings—pioneers in the field of artificial organs like Belding Scribner, Carl Kjellstrand, Michael DeBakey, Willem J. Kolff, and Pierre Galletti—were once again on the program, but they talked about things that had seldom come up before. They talked—and argued—about whether there should be limits on what we do to extend life, about whether high-technology medical care should be available to people regardless of race and economic class, about whether we have overspent on medical care, and about whether technology had all the answers.

Viewed in retrospect, the discussion that morning can be seen as a manifestation of the beginning of an inexorable change in the focus of those who have spent their professional careers in biomedical engineering. Medical and biological engineers must now confront a set of issues and questions that most have not been trained to consider. If they do not engage these questions constructively, they, and everyone else, will find themselves forced to live with the consequences of allowing others to do that work. That is why this book is so important. Chapter 1 presented a medical perspective on these questions. This chapter approaches them from an engineering point of view, placing them in the broader context of the general tension in society regarding public policy in its relation to technology.

Biomedical engineers have generally become involved with medical and biological engineering because of their fascination with the challenge of linking the physical sciences and engineering with biology and medicine. There is a satisfaction, almost aesthetic in nature, in creative problem-solving that brings together previously disparate disciplines such as physiology, chemical engineering, materials science, instrumentation, and design. In the developmental stages of the field, professionals in one discipline learned to talk to professionals in other disciplines. Physical scientists and engineers learned to explain the relevance of their work to medical scientists; researchers learned to deal with clinicians. Professionals were both "suppliers" and "consumers," funding was fairly plentiful, and both the effort and the outcome were satisfying.

These were conditions that existed in a number of technical fields in the United States in the post-World War II era and especially since the launching of Sputnik in 1957. In fact, Jean-Claude Derian, former Chief Science Counselor at the French Embassy in Washington, in his recent book *America's Struggle for Leadership in Technology*[2] argued that these conditions had given rise to a "sheltered technological culture" in the United States. It was one characterized by assured markets; what we invented would be used. Agencies or industries were willing to make commitments to the major up-front costs of technological development. Engineering optimization could be based on quality and performance, not on cost or need. Our strategy was one of "technology push" rather than "societal pull"—what we developed and marketed was whatever engineering ingenuity could create.

That bubble, as Derian notes, is bursting in this country in many fields and for many different reasons. It burst for AT&T with deregulation, which thrust them into a competitive environment that was completely unfamiliar to them. It has taken that company years to adjust and it is only now learning how to function in our new world. It happened to those in the semiconductor industry when they discovered that industrial leadership was not only a function of good technical ideas but also depended on productive and efficient manufacturing and aggressive marketing. It happened in the field of nuclear power when scientists and engineers encountered the social fear and unacceptability of their product. And it is now happening in biomedical engineering, where it is equally traumatic.

The causes of the disruption in the case of biomedical engineering are a confluence of social realities—the "externalities" of our field—that can no longer be ignored. They reflect, first of all, social needs and problems. The U.S. has medically under-served many populations—minorities, those who live in rural communities, the uninsured. Infant mortality and life expectancy figures are not what one would expect in a developed country that claims a role of global leadership. On the other hand, there are serious economic constraints at work in the United States which require that the society set priorities for its expenditures.

In setting priorities, however, we must confront and deal with the ethical imperatives in the delivery of medical care. The principles of biomedical ethics include respect for the dignity and autonomy of the individual, commitment to beneficence—that is, to do no harm to people—and attention to distributive justice. Each impinges on biomedicine and each introduces subtleties of interpretation about which people of goodwill can disagree, but even these do not exhaust the social issues with which we need to be concerned. Beyond needs, economics, and ethics, the work of biomedical engineers is affected by a society's cultural values—in a sense, its prejudices.

One obvious manifestation of these culturally defined values is the distinction between objective risk—generally, a quantifiable notion—and risk perception. How people perceive risk, and how they approach its management, is very much a function of how they view technology: technophiles who believe—perhaps too strongly—in technical solutions to all problems tend to understate risk; technophobes, who want nothing to do with technology, tend to overstate it. Although it is true that most people fall between these two extremes, biomedical engineers must face the present reality that, where the human body is concerned, American society tends toward the technophobic point of view.

Consider, for example, the reaction that most people would have to the novel medical management of a previously fatal disease in which a physician was able to achieve a 90 percent cure rate but actively contributed to the death of the other 10 percent. It is likely that the vast majority of people would view this as a medical breakthrough, a great accomplishment. Compare that with the likely response to a machine that did the same thing—saved 90 percent and killed 10 percent. Although there is no data to support the conclusion, most of us would expect the reaction in this case to be negative and the litigation vigorous. To most people, there is something dehumanizing about technology; and to the extent that society is alienated from technology, it will hold it to a much higher standard with respect to risk.

Social needs, economics, ethics, and cultural prejudices, taken in aggregate, represent the unstructured, but nevertheless real, interests that manifest themselves in the actions governments take to influence the development and adoption of technology in medicine. Also, in our society, government "action" has its own set of characteristics with which the biomedical engineering community must contend: first, it is primarily regulatory in nature, aimed at establishing controls rather than incentives or guidance; second, it is usually focused on the process rather than the outcome; third, it is concerned with time scales that are very much shorter than those usually associated with technological development, a mismatch, in feedback control terms, that is highly likely to lead to instabilities.

Finally, biomedical engineers, fairly or unfairly, are burdened with a responsibility that arises from how others use their products: the companies that sell them, the hospitals that buy them, the clinicians who use them.

None of these externalities represents a well-defined issue: they are interpreted differently by different people; they shift in relative importance over time; they are not easily quantifiable. Moreover, they are not independent problems; they interact in various ways. Although engineers are used to dealing with complicated realities and finding ways to model and cope with them, the familiar complications of physical phenomena are far different from those of social phenomena. A common and understandable reaction to the new circumstances that have burst the bubble of our version of Derian's "sheltered technological culture" is frustration. These new problems are not ones that we like and not ones that we believe to be our fair burden. Frustration, however, is not a productive stimulus to effective action. This is our new reality, and our ability and willingness to cope with problems we don't like may well determine how free we will be to work on the problems that first attracted us to this field as well as how successful we will be in contributing to health care.

The remainder of this chapter is devoted to a discussion of some of these new problems to illustrate some aspects of their complexity and some ways of thinking about them. It will begin with what must be a much longer and comprehensive effort to find ways of incorporating these social constraints into our own efforts, where that is appropriate, and of explaining ourselves and our field to others, where that is necessary.

* * * *

We begin with economic issues, since the crisis in the cost of medical care has been a major driving force in raising people's sensitivity to technology in medicine. Technology has certainly contributed to medical costs, although its contribution is often exaggerated. It is difficult to get accurate data, but some estimates have indicated that about 25 percent of health costs (and of health cost increases) are associated with technology, suggesting, of course, that 75 percent arises from other factors.

With respect to technology-connected costs, it is important to keep in mind the difference between unit costs and aggregate costs. These are illustrated in the four examples shown in Table 1. Kidney dialysis costs about $25,000 per patient per year. The impact, however, is not in the unit cost; it is that, with 120,000 patients kept alive through this therapy, the total cost is $3 billion a year, or about 0.4 percent of our total national health care bill for 0.05 percent of our population.

On the other hand, heart transplants, which cost about $300,000 per patient, are limited by organ availability to about 2,000 per year. Thus, even if we placed no restrictions on transplant reimbursement, the total cost to the nation would be only about $600 million annually. This is still a large number, but it is much smaller than the cost of dialysis, and it is not likely to get much larger. In this case, the issue is not one of opening the floodgates to huge aggregate costs for this therapy, but whether we consider it "worthwhile" to spend $300,000—the unit cost—on individual patients; that is, do we consider it cost-effective? There is, of course, a non-financial issue as well: the question of equity—who gets transplants and who doesn't. That becomes an even more difficult question if public reimbursement systems don't cover heart transplants while private systems do, and a scarce resource is thus distributed not on the basis of need or optimal benefit but on the basis of the patient's financial capacity.

Table 1
UNIT vs. AGGREGATE COSTS

Kidney Dialysis
    $25,000/patient/yr × 120,000 patients = $3 billion/yr

Heart Transplants
    $298,200/patient × 2,000 patients/yr = $0.6 billion/yr

Artificial Hearts
    $328,000/patient × 35,000 patients/yr = $11.5 billion/yr

CVS Scans
    $1,000/scan × 500 p./D.S. case = $500,000/D.S. case

According to current estimates, the artificial heart, when it is finally available, will cost about $330,000 per patient.[3] However, here there is no natural limitation on the availability of artificial hearts and, with up to 70,000 people who might benefit from the heart, the total cost to society could reach $20 billion or more, clearly a matter of great concern. This has led a number of people to argue that we should abandon efforts to complete this development because the clinical costs would be too high. On the other hand, let us assume that a vigorous anti-smoking campaign over the next few decades could reduce the incidence of end-stage heart disease to a much smaller number, perhaps 3,000 to 4,000 per year. Would (or should) the artificial heart then become more acceptable to society?

The final example illustrates a different aspect of the distinction between unit and aggregate cost. CVS scans are performed on pregnant women above a certain age to detect any of a number of diseases, but primarily Down's Syndrome. For illustrative purposes, assume that it costs about $1,000 per scan and that about one in 500 scans reveals a fetus with Down's Syndrome. That would mean that we spend $500,000 for each case of Down's Syndrome uncovered. As we move toward applying cost-effectiveness criteria to priorities in medical treatment, how shall we judge such a procedure? One of the things we may want to consider is what we can or should do with the information. For instance, if a fetus with Down's Syndrome is aborted, then it might be reasonable to weigh the $500,000 cost involved in identifying it against the cost to society of a lifetime of care for a person with that condition. However, if that is to be the nature of the calculation, should we then limit

CVS scans to those women committed to choosing abortion if a Down's Syndrome fetus is identified? Clearly, economic decisions are tightly interwoven with a number of social and ethical issues.

The cost to the health care system of technology-based care arises not only from the cost of the technology itself but also from the social system into which it is introduced. The litigiousness of our society leads to what is sometimes called "defensive medical practices," erring on the side of more rather than less use of sophisticated treatments to avoid negligence suits, and thereby incurring costs that can far exceed those directly related to lawsuits.

Competition in medical care, unlike in many other fields, may actually raise costs instead of reducing them. When the strategy for improving one's competitive position is to provide an impressive range of sophisticated and expensive equipment, everyone pays for the excess capacity either through its unnecessary use or through increased fees. When hospitals performing only a few transplants per year advertise themselves as transplant centers, everyone pays for the overhead of maintaining transplant teams (or for the poor results that come from insufficient experience).

Although all expenses are real, not all are unreasonable, nor ought we to feel apologetic about them. For example, if a technology is introduced for treating a disease not previously treatable, medical expenses will go up because we are able to treat more people, not because we have introduced inherently expensive medicine. The new treatment of the new disease may, in fact, be more cost-effective in saving lives than existing treatments of *other* diseases. In such cases, if total costs are to be controlled, the sensible approach would be to phase out existing treatments that are less cost-effective. As the Oregon experience has indicated, there are grave practical difficulties in implementing such regulatory systems; but biomedical engineers should be thinking about how they might contribute to that effort.

There are several other ways in which the biomedical engineering community can contribute to the effort to control health care costs and to the dialogue about that effort. With respect to the control of costs, we must move beyond the "technology push" mentality: cost must become as important a criterion as performance in a new product; need must become as important as feasibility in undertaking a new development; the goal of reducing total health care costs must drive our efforts as much as the goal of increasing the potential for treating disease.

With respect to the dialogue about cost control, we must familiarize decision-makers with the nature of technology. For example, they must begin to understand the technology learning curve: that the cost of a given technology always decreases and its effectiveness increases over time. Therefore cost-effectiveness comparisons made at the time of introduction of a technology will always be misleading. If adverse decisions are made on the basis of that initial comparison, the ultimate benefit will be lost. As another example, decision-makers and the public at large must be helped to understand the highly nonlinear costs of reliability. No technology is risk free, and when society insists upon reductions in risk potential to unrealistically low levels, it raises unit costs so high that the effectiveness of health care is actually reduced. That is, there are opportunity costs associated with risk reduction: increasing system reliability from 90 percent to 99 percent may help 9 percent of the treated population, but the increased cost may mean that a vastly larger number of people will not be treated at all. Can the biomedical engineering community help to promote societal acceptance of a more realistic approach to risk?

* * * *

Most public discussion of medical technologies has concerned their economic impact. However, there are many other dimensions to their social impact and each deserves attention. In the following paragraphs, a number of examples are presented, not in any attempt to be comprehensive or exhaustive, but rather to illustrate the range of issues.

The term "medical technology" is applied to a wide range of rather disparate systems that draw on many different kinds of technologies of varying levels of sophistication and are applied to many different aspects of the health care system. There is no easy or precise way to systematically categorize these many systems but, for some purposes, it is convenient to divide them into those that are used for diagnosis and those that are used for therapy. Generally speaking, the diagnostic systems depend heavily on information technologies—signal acquisition and processing, as well as the manipulation and storage of information—drawing on the skills of electrical engineers, physicists, and computer scientists. Therapeutic systems, on the other hand, tend to depend on disciplines such as molecular biology, biochemistry, materials science, and transport phenomena, and their direct intervention in the body's functioning gives rise to greater concerns about reliability and quality of life. Genetic analysis, "smart" monitors, and patient databases are three examples of diagnostic technologies, each rather different from the others. Genetically engineered drugs, dialysis, and artificial hearts are examples of therapeutic technologies, also different from each other.

• **Genetic analysis** has not only been extremely important in research aimed at identifying and correcting genetic defects but also it has made it possible to identify latent disease conditions sufficiently early that options are available to deal with them. Down's Syndrome is certainly one example, but there are now many others. However, the very effectiveness of these methods has become a source of social concern, frequently cast in terms of the competing claims of individual privacy and the public good. Who ought to have access to this information? Should individuals be stigmatized because they are known to have a certain trait? Should there be any public right to information about an individual or a family in a world where employers and insurance companies have begun to take very seriously the issue of risk management? Should prospective parents have a right to information about a fetus that might lead them to choose to abort it for reasons that might range from the questionable to the frivolous—wrong sex, high risk for certain diseases? Indeed, is it possible that the very ability to identify and possibly correct certain problems *in utero* raises the specter of eugenics and changes perceptions about the worth of "defective" people? All of these issues are now being raised by bioethicists and public interest groups.

• **"Smart" monitors** raise a quite different set of issues. These devices, associated with such systems as implantable defibrillators or glucose pumps, not only monitor vital signals continuously but can initiate actions in response to those signals, thus offering a patient a level of care that approaches having a physician continuously present. But an instrument is not a physician, and society's view of liability is quite different with respect to a machine than it is with respect to a human being. If we are to gain the advantages that could come from wider use of these new monitors, we must deal intelligently with these legal issues.

• **Data bases,** which may have the greatest potential for reducing medical costs of any single kind of technology, have had surprisingly little use in medical care. Information technology is now being widely applied in field after field, in business after business. The private sector is investing heavily in it because it is found to be economical—it saves companies money and gives them quick information useful for managing. Interestingly, however, where information exchange crosses the boundaries of individual companies (or practitioners), or where it requires a public investment in data networks, it is used much less often. The sharing of medical information is certainly inhibited by the lack of these networks and there seems to be little impetus to change things. Physicians and hospitals aren't too eager automatically to share information on patients and patients aren't too eager to have it floating around, particularly because of the current business strategy of insurance companies. Physicians—unlike lawyers—take little advantage of the potential for continuing medical education or treatment updates that an information network could provide, probably because there is no way to obtain reimbursement for the investment in the technology. So, while this is a technology whose increased use would certainly lower medical costs and would probably improve care, we don't seem to have a social organizational structure that can bring about its adoption.

• **Genetically engineered drugs,** such as tissue plasminogen activator and erythropoietin, have sensitized us to the difficult problem of finding equitable approaches to making drugs available to the public at a reasonable cost while allowing drug companies to recoup the enormous research and development costs associated with new drugs. Particularly in this area, the more general societal question of "industrial policy" looms large. A tension has developed between governmental attempts to simplify the drug approval process on the one hand (lowering development costs, but raising concerns about safety issues) and, on the other hand, granting increased intellectual property protection to companies through such mechanisms as the Orphan Drug Act (with its attendant potential for windfall profits). The extension of patent protection to the life-forms used to manufacture these drugs has also raised an issue that had great prominence in the discussion of the treaty on biodiversity at the United Nations Conference on Environment and Development at Rio de Janeiro in 1992. The nations of the developing world argued that the patenting of life-forms has established a precedent for abandoning the long-established tradition that a nation is not entitled to compensation for the products developed from germ plasm obtained and removed from its territory.

• **Artificial organs** is an imprecise term used to refer to devices or systems that replace some or all of the functions of a natural organ. It could include, for example, dialysis machines and membrane oxygenators as well as artificial hearts. What they have in common is that they don't cure a disease but help people to live with it over the course of their lives. As a consequence, quality of life emerges as a major issue, and with respect to implanted devices reliable functioning over periods of time that may extend to five, ten, or even twenty years is an important performance criterion. Both present major problems. With respect to quality of life, who ought to make the judgment? With respect to performance, how shall we define it, how high a standard should we set, and how shall we demonstrate, in realistic timeframes, that a system or device can meet our expectations? Moreover, how should we compare the outcomes achievable using these devices with those achievable with existing therapies—that is, how do we establish relative cost-effectiveness?

The reports of the last few advisory groups called upon to assess progress in the NHLBI's artificial heart program have begun to deal with these issues,[3] introducing a measure termed quality adjusted life years (QALY). To calculate QALY, the extended years of life achieved by a certain therapy is multiplied by a "quality of life parameter," a number between zero and one that represents a quantitative representation of some qualitative judgment of how "normal"/good/pleasant a person's life is as a result of the therapy. If the cost of the therapy is factored in, one can calculate a cost-effectiveness measure—QALY/dollar spent.

Table 2 illustrates the use of this approach to compare conventional treatment for end-stage heart disease with that for heart transplantation and with the projected costs of the artificial heart. As the table shows, by this measure the most cost-effective procedure is a transplant. Perhaps surprisingly, the least cost-effective procedure is the conventional drug treatment, not only because patients only survive for six months on average but also because the accompanying extremely limited "bed-to-chair" existence is assigned a very low quality of life parameter. The table demonstrates an important point sometimes lost in the public discussion of whether or not to introduce "expensive" therapies: although the cost-effectiveness of artificial hearts is still lower than that of heart transplants, and though our health dollars might be better spent for other purposes, consistency of reasoning would dictate that we ought to *stop* providing conventional treatment to heart patients because that is still less effective.

Table 2
END-STAGE HEART DISEASE:
COST-EFFECTIVENESS OF THERAPIES

Therapy	Aggregate Cost (K$)	Life-Years (years)	QALY (years)
Conventional Treatment	28.5	0.50	0.03
Transplantation	298.2	11.30	8.45
Artificial Heart	327.6	4.42	2.88

Thus, two significant issues are raised. First, it makes little sense to argue that the way to hold down medical costs is to limit or halt the introduction of new technologies; in fact, we might actually reduce costs in circumstances in which new technologies are more cost-effective. Second, cost-effectiveness as a concept has some serious limitations in terms of the values of the society. Are we really prepared to halt conventional treatment of heart patients based only on an economic argument? The Oregon experience indicates how wrenching such an approach is to society. There are many who believe that the Oregon plan will not be broadly emulated within the United States. As rational as the approach may be, until there are significant changes in the attitudes of people about life and death, about how to define their own humanity and humaneness, rationality and cost-effectiveness will not be viewed as the exclusive criteria for judging the delivery of health care.

It would be a mistake, however, to reach the conclusion that new technology is always more cost-effective and, even more important, that making it so is accepted as a major obligation. Generally speaking, the sheltered technological culture which we have inherited has not inculcated that as a major motivation. For example, during the years in which dialysis has been covered by Medicare, its costs have remained approximately equal to the government's payment schedule. Home dialysis costs have actually increased over those years to reach that schedule. Interestingly, the cost of a disposable dialyzing unit has gone down during that time, as one would expect. Surely, dialysis is safer today than it once was, and it is probably more effective, but it is not cheaper. Clearly, cost reduction has not been a goal; one of the challenges to the biomedical community is to change that situation.

* * * *

To conclude, we return to where we began. Scientists and engineers committed to the application of technology to problems in medicine must deal not only with the challenging complexities of biological systems; they must also recognize the equally complex realities of human society with its political, social, cultural, and religious values and structures. As with any highly interactive system, a disturbance in one part has consequences throughout. To the extent that those involved in the development of technology can anticipate these many interactions, they can work constructively to help society to deal with them. In a sense, what is needed is the social equivalent of an environmental impact statement. If the engineers who best understand these new systems take the lead in objectively assessing them, they will be in a better position to insure that the assessment is an informed one.

References

1. *ASAIO Transactions*, 35(3), 1989.

2. J.-C. Derian, *America's Struggle for Leadership in Technology* (Cambridge: MIT Press, 1990).

3. J.R. Hogness and M. Van Antwerp, eds., *The Artificial Heart: Prototypes, Policies, and Patients* (Washington, D.C.: National Academy Press, 1991).

CHAPTER 3

A View from the Senate

DAVID DURENBERGER
U.S. Senator, Minnesota

"A dysfunctional medical market system is depriving us of the resources we need...to serve the *real* health needs of the people."

"Fourteen percent of our GNP is currently going into medical 'solutions' to long-term health care *failure*."

"Solving the problem involves...changing our values."

Washington is attempting to solve a problem which has not yet been defined. In 1988 the major health care issue was long-term care. A recommendation on long-term care was put on the shelf and has not been pulled off in the last three years. Acute care has not been perceived as a political problem. A problem that *was* perceived was that there were 36 million uninsured Americans. The issue of cost of access was not even addressed in the three years preceding September 1990. Today, both parties, Democrats and Republicans, have coalesced around some of the realities that face the American people. They want high-quality care, but the cost of access to that care is a problem. The problem of job loss has health care loss connected with it. In one way or another, cost has become a large part of the problem.

One problem for Americans is our *definition* of health, health care, and health policy. We have "medicalized" those definitions. A real challenge in America is to broaden the definition of health to include the behavioral and other problems we see around us. The drive-by shootings, the kids killing each other for sneakers—these are a large part of this problem. Medical access also is a part of that problem. Long-term access to long-term care is also a part of that problem. The environment should be part of health policy in this country; genetics is part of health policy in this country.

One of the things we ought to emulate is the way other major countries define health. Almost all of them define it in this much larger context. Only in America have we totally "medicalized" the definition of health care. Today our fetish for medical solutions and our dysfunctional medical market system are depriving us of the resources we need for the family, the community, and the country to serve the *real* health needs of the people. Fourteen percent of our GNP is currently going into medical "solutions" to long-term health care *failure*.

Solving the problem involves cost containment. It also involves changing our values. Americans want the job security of having health insurance; they want costs under control or at least predictable; they want high-quality care. They don't want to stand in lines; they don't want second-rate medicine. This in effect means that most Americans want more and better for less.

How can we meet that challenge? It can be met politically by turning the whole system over to the government, or a market approach can be found to resolve the problem. I don't know of any particular public service in which turning over a problem to the government has worked—in which you need more and better but you want to pay less. Government productivity is an oxymoron.

Many of my friends insist that the solution is mandated pay or play—employer mandates must cover everybody on the existing system. In my opinion, that is not going to do it. Others propose a single-payer solution and want all states to do what Canada does. But if America turns its system into a Canadian-style system, where are Canadians going to get their medical care?

The way to do more and better for less is to increase *productivity*. It means we have to change the behavior of everybody in the current system. We as consumers have to change, producers and providers of care have to change, and the health plans which provide us access have to change as well. Employers have to change their behavior and the government has to become more productive. Wherever you look in this particular system, you have to find ways to do better at less cost. The best way to restrain cost growth is to improve quality.

Among my many constituencies is the Mayo Clinic. The Mayo Clinic is running out of business. If it is the best in the world, why is it running out of business? It has a thousand doctors and a thousand residents, and it is running out of work. So don't tell me Americans know how to buy quality medical care. We ought to be lined up in front of the Mayo Clinic instead of our local hospitals. But we aren't because we don't know any better.

Improving and defining quality is critical. The debate presently being waged includes the managed-competition people on one side and the regulators on the other. In effect what we have is an issue in which cost-containment is one side of the policy debate and coverage is the other side. On the cost-containment side, it is my view that the only way to contain costs is to reward the best producers in our system with *all* of the business. In order to do this, we have to be able to reward the consumers of health care with dollar savings when they buy the right kind of health plans that give them access to the right kind of medical services. That is the essence of managed competition.

Employers, *not* the government, are doing this right now in my home state. Employers in my state over the last ten to twelve years have found ways through HMOs and other kinds of accountable health plans to reduce the cost of health care in Minnesota from 10 percent above the national average to 15 percent below the national average. In Rochester health care cost is 23 percent below the national average; in Los Angeles, it is 78 percent above the national average. If everybody in America did what we are doing in Minnesota—changing the way medicine is practiced, changing the way people buy their health care—we would probably have our health care costs back at 9 percent or 10 percent of the GNP within a decade. The key is rewarding good providers for their good behavior and letting them show us what good behavior is. Let them show us what the most appropriate use of technology is and what kind of technology we really need.

We are just beginning this process. Minneapolis-St. Paul has a population of 2.1 million people, and we have *closed* the equivalent of ten 400-bed hospitals over the last ten years. The hospitals that remain are operating at only 46 percent of capacity. Similar things can be done a market at a time all over America.

The coverage side is where the Clinton administration has some problems. They want to reform coverage and do market reform at the same time, and I don't believe you can do that. In order to make a market work, the consumers have to get the financial rewards. In order to make a market work, I have to get some savings by choosing the better health plan. By doing the correct and responsible thing for my health I have to see a benefit which is not ripped off by somebody in the system. Most of the savings in a market need to go to the person who makes the market work—the consumer.

It is very important that we look elsewhere for universal coverage. The elsewhere is already there—the federal subsidies for employer-paid health insurance, tax subsidies for our own illnesses, Medicaid, Medicare, the VA, and retiree health benefits. There is sufficient money in the system right now that, if it were spent more appropriately, it could provide universal coverage. Why is it that at age 65 we make everybody change the way they buy health protection? We subsidize the big companies, the well-off, and the rich, and we penalize the self-employed and individuals in small groups.

There is so much room for change. This is one of those times when the solution is in all of us. It takes a leader like Bill Clinton and a leader like Hillary Rodham Clinton to give us the vision for the future of American health care and create a truly American solution to our nation's number-one challenge.

CHAPTER 4

A View from
Several Perspectives

GAIL WILENSKY
Project Hope

"There is nothing like a problem becoming a middle-class problem to move it up on the political agenda."

"Everything about the way we have arranged health care now encourages people to want more, provide more, consume more, and spend more on health care.... Our tax system encourages people to take a lot of health insurance rather than higher wages."

"We have not had much incentive to adopt cost-reducing technologies.... We need to reward cost-reducing technologies and to provide incentives to use them where they count."

"We must accomplish...these major goals...without destroying the incentives for innovation and change and high quality."

"The real potential for the future is in bioengineering."

Why are we hearing so much about health care reform today? Because we have 36 million people who are uninsured? Because we keep spending two to three times more on health care than we do on other things? No. The reason we are so concerned about health care reform now has more to do with the fact that the recession of 1990 was a white-collar recession. Middle-class people who had not previously been worried about health care and health insurance realized that people like themselves were losing their jobs and, with their jobs, their insurance. Because of the strange way health insurance works, even if those people regained employment, they might not be able to get insurance due to an illness or a preexisting condition. Thus, a problem that has existed for more than thirty years became a real middle-class problem. There is nothing like a problem becoming a middle-class problem to move it up on the political agenda.

Those of us in public policy positions are, on the other hand, more worried about rising national health expenditures and the numbers of people without insurance. You are hearing many schizophrenic responses as to what problem we are trying to face. Both sets of problems are out there: the problems *individuals* tend to think about, which are, "How can I reduce the costs that I face?" or "How can I make sure that *my* health care and *my* health insurance is stable and there when I need it?" and the questions our politicians are concerned about, such as "How can we make sure that health care is provided to people who have been shut out of the system?" Even more important, from the politicians' point of view, is the question, "How can we begin to restrain health care spending?" These two perspectives are not always the same, and they are going to cause a lot of problems.

Let me now share with you the roles that technology and biomedical engineering can play, although I don't think they have always played these roles in the past. There is no question that many people in this country attribute a part, sometimes a large part, of our health care cost problem to spending on technology—its use and its misuse. We should not be surprised that spending is an issue in this country—everything about the way we have arranged health care now encourages people to want more, provide more, consume more, and spend more on health care, and that certainly extends to the area of health care technology. The question is, "How are we going to address this spending concern?" What sorts of methods are we going to adopt to slow spending, and what will such restraints mean for health care technological innovation and for biomedical engineering? We must address these issues adequately if we wish to avoid severe damage to the system.

It is no real surprise that this is a problem. Typically, consumers are shielded from the cost of health care. That is part of what it means to have health insurance, and constitutes both the good and the bad of health insurance. Our tax system encourages people to take a lot of health insurance rather than higher wages in their employee compensation packages. We have numerous structures that encourage physicians and institutions to use any procedure that might provide some medical benefit, even if there is some real question about whether the benefit provided is anywhere comparable to its costs, either to the individual institution or to society as a whole. The incentive for such action is partly the reimbursement system, partly the liability system. If a physician or institution doesn't do anything and everything that someone else might have done in those circumstances, and the patient has a bad outcome, then the individual and the institution will be subject to a lawsuit. If we are going to moderate spending, we are going to have to find ways to change the incentives motivating consumers, providers of health care, individual physicians, and institutions, and we must also reform our concepts of liability.

Many of our health policy colleagues have joined the camp of those who feel that technology has been a real cost-driver, that technology is so powerful a cost-driver that if we do not severely and harshly restrain the introduction and/or diffusion of new technology, we will not be able to control spending—even if it is technology for which people want to spend money. That is frightening. It is politically unrealistic to adopt a position that even if people understood what a specific technology costs and thought it worthwhile we should not allow it to be applied. The fact that a number of my colleagues indeed feel this way distresses me.

Let me share with you the reasons why I don't have this fear. When people understand the cost implication of new technology being used well (however we define that), if they know, understand, and acknowledge that there is a price to be paid for what the technology could bring, we ought to provide it. This is not a danger. In the past we have not had much incentive to adopt cost-reducing technologies, and we have not had much incentive to use technologies in places where they really make sense from a cost point-of-view. Our incentives have pushed us to adopt any technology that provides *any* new medical benefit, *period*. These incentives spring from the structure of the reimbursement system. Reimbursement is typically provided on a cost basis, with the cost being passed through to insurance companies. This is the basic reason why it is only in health care that technology has *not* resulted in cost-reducing strategies. In most other areas of endeavor technology is looked to as a way to provide more things or better things more cheaply. Why is that not the case in health care? Two reasons:

- there is no direct incentive for providing cost-reducing technologies;
- there is very little incentive to use such technologies because of our reimbursement system.

We need to reward cost-reducing technologies and to provide incentives to use them where they count. There are very few technologies that are not cost-reducing some of the time. The argument should not be whether, on a unit basis, they reduce cost. Yes, it is cheaper to do angioplasty than it is to do bypass surgery. Yes, it is cheaper to do some sophisticated imaging, even if it is very expensive, than to do some expensive invasive surgery. However, it is not cheaper *for the system* if five or ten times as many people have angioplasty or imaging procedures as would have had surgery. These procedures are only worthwhile if their use is determined at the level of the individual patient; that is, if the technology is used with discretion. What we need, therefore, is both better knowledge about what works and when, and a reimbursement system that supports doing things when they count. I very much agree with Thier (see Chapter 1) that it is not just cost in the narrow sense that we want to examine, but costs in the overall sense.

The question is, can we begin to find ways to provide financial incentives to develop cost-reducing technologies rather than just anything that provides any benefit? And can we find ways to encourage their use when it counts? Achieving these goals will require a change from the way we do things now. The initial obstacle is a lack of information about what works, although there is increased interest in outcomes research and on making that information available. Presently there are not financial incentives to use cost-reducing technologies or to develop them; that needs to change. There are no incentives to do things when they count most rather than simply providing procedures for everyone.

We should be worried about health care reform. It is not just a matter of trying to make sure that we find a way to provide health insurance coverage to the people who are now without it, or to find a way to moderate spending. We must accomplish both of these major goals at the same time without destroying the incentives for innovation and change and the high quality of health care that American consumers of health care for so long have taken for granted. It is not an easy order. Don't be fooled by people who claim it is. It will require very delicate trade-offs if we are to achieve the goals of decreased cost and increased access without killing the drive for innovation and change that has so distinguished the American health care system.

The real potential for the future is in bioengineering. The desire for new knowledge and better ways of doing things is so much an inherent part of our society that, in the end, I believe the good sense of our American citizens will prevail.

CHAPTER 5

Public Policy and Innovation

SUSAN BARTLETT FOOTE

"The support structure for basic science and technology must relate and correlate to social needs. . . . We have used payment policy as the implicit technology policy."

"Most politicians do not have the appropriate skills . . . for technological decisions."

"We need input . . . in the area of emerging technologies that . . . may have great benefit. . . . Medical and biological engineers are the people who know what the new emerging technologies might be."

"Technology is not simply a cost problem. It is a health care quality issue."

Only an academic thinks coming to Washington is coming to the real world. Washington has its own form of virtual reality. We have a technology policy challenge; now is the time to develop the solution. We now have the opportunity to come up with a new medical technology policy. The problem is that technology issues are complex, hard to understand, and not well understood in the policy environment. Technology is often treated in the debate as an after-thought, an add-on, something separate from health reform. It is something to worry about, to be ambivalent about, to blame for cost increases when it is convenient to do so. Both the public and the policymakers are not very well informed about the tremendous complexity and interrelation of technology to all aspects of health care.

Health policy planners need help in order to do their job right. If we do it wrong, it will cause tremendous damage not just to you professionally, but to the quality of our health care for decades to come.

The stages of innovation are presented in Figure 1. Note that in medical technology, unlike other areas of technology innovation, government and public policy have become imbedded in the innovative process at virtually every stage. In terms of support of innovation, a large number of government agencies are involved, including the NIH, NSF, DOD, and NASA. There are private-sector pressures on the innovative process as well. Virtually everywhere there is some kind of government agency that gets involved with either pushing that technology, to use Keller's term (Chapter 2), or pulling it back and inhibiting it in some way. I have described these various public policies, where they came from, what they do, and how they change.[1]

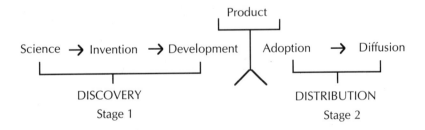

Figure 1. The Stages of Innovation.

There is very little interchange in Washington among these various sources of public policy. When we consider changing the incentives in public policy, we must deal with entrenched bureaucracies with lives of their own that operate in ways very much independent of each other. One of the big challenges, if we are really to have a rational medical technology policy, is to redesign the federal bureaucracy. The support structure for basic science and technology must relate and correlate to social needs; there must be some feedback between the two. That is one challenge. Considering the health reform to date, our technology policy, to the extent that we have one, is really our payment policy. We have used payment policy as the implicit technology policy. When we talk about health reform and attempt to redesign the structure, focusing primarily on payment and cost, we are indeed implicitly designing a not very well understood technology policy.

There is considerable uncertainty about what exactly will come out of the Clinton White House. There are really two paradigms at far ends of the spectrum that are possible models—public regulation or managed competition. Health reform most likely will fall somewhere within those paradigms (Figure 2).

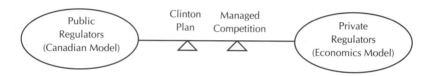

Figure 2. The Spectrum of Health Reform Paradigms.

On the *public regulator* side, government must make fundamental decisions; the source of public policy will be government—and government means politics. If you have ever tried to discuss EKG-reimbursement policy with a senator for hours because that is the pressing issue of the day, and this is someone who has never given an EKG or designed an EKG device, you realize that politicians do not have the appropriate skills and should not be required to micromanage technology decisions. The minute there is government there is politics, and the minute there is politics there are other factors and biases that come into play.

The *managed competition model* relies primarily on the private sector to regulate the marketplace—competition among health plans will be the cost-control mechanism, not a price-setting government entity. It is a model that is driven primarily by economics rather than politics.

The preference of conservative Democrats and moderate Republicans, which I support, is to design technology policy as part of the economic or private-sector regulatory side. Some, however, only give lip service to the competitive model. What may develop is a design that looks much more like a public regulator than a private economic system. That can be done in a number of ways. Most congressional staffers haven't spent ten years in a business school, so they don't always understand or trust markets. They think in terms of government, because that is what they know. Government means making rules and regulations, with punishments for violators. A big danger is that we will have a program that is *called* managed competition but really isn't. What may happen is that government will make the technology policy in-house. First, you will get centralization—the federal system making decisions about technologies for the whole country, not just for Medicare, not just for Medicaid, but for privately insured persons as well. What is the government's track record? On both technology assessment and on coverage and payment policy it is pretty dismal. There are technologies buried in the morass of HCFA. There are delays and bureaucracy. Government tends to undervalue assessment—it isn't a service for which we pay very much. One percent of health care spending goes to government assessment activities, a very small investment in assessment.

If we go to a price regulation model, we get into a problem Dr. Weisbrod raised (Chapter 10). If the price is set wrong, then the technology can be lost because all the signals say to the manufacturer or provider that they will lose money. It doesn't take very long for hospitals and other providers to decide that they simply cannot get involved in a technology that will lose money every time. There is a tremendous danger that addressing cost containment by centralization is going to paralyze technology. Government is not good at picking winners and losers and is not good at pricing them.

There is a lot more promise on the private regulator side. Weisbrod (Chapter 10) has discussed the insurance issues. We are not going to go to a system where fewer people are covered; we are going to keep an insurance system, and we need to restructure the insurance market so that the incentives to overutilize and overconsume are changed. The efforts to create capitated, HMO-like, accountable health plans, not based on a fee-for-service model, are important. Putting the risks of the health of the covered individuals in the hands of the insurance provider in an integrated system means that there is much less incentive to overutilize care and much greater incentive for rational allocation of high-cost capital equipment. I have been accused of saying "Americans like to bury the hard decisions in the private sector." That is how it should be. Health plans are going to be measured on outcomes rather than on inputs. It is not how many MRIs a particular plan has, but how well the patients do in that plan. This will be the information by which consumers make selections, thus depoliticizing much of the decision making.

Where problems still lie, and where we need input, is in the area of emerging technologies that may be cost-raising locally or in the short term but that still may have great benefit. We need some incentives for greater assessment and understanding of the value of those technologies. The challenge is to design a federal role that doesn't just block emerging technologies but builds in incentives for the private sector to cooperate with the public sector to provide the kind of information we need to understand just what it is that these technologies might contribute, and to encourage them if we need greater understanding. We also need a mechanism or process by which we can move from the innovative stage through the experimental stage to the decision to adopt the technology. There are some technologies that won't be buried in the private sector, because the issues are not merely those of cost effectiveness. The private sector can do cost-effectiveness measures pretty well. There are some technologies which the public will perceive as a treatment and, assuming it will be a benefit to them, will insist that it be included in the benefit package. As long as there is some kind of standard benefit package, there is going to be tremendous pressure for the federal government to have some system of making decisions about the values of those new technologies.

That is where we really need help—because medical and biological engineers are the people who know what the new emerging technologies might be and who they can help. We don't want to lose the momentum in the R&D sector, which is at risk of being lost if we are not careful. Technology is not simply a cost problem; it is a health care quality issue. Bring information to help those of us who are working on this problem do a better job. It is in my interest, your interest, and society's interest to do so.

Discussion

In response to a question dealing with incentives and the production of physicians, Dr. Foote said: "There is as much as $30 billion in the Medicare system for reimbursement for GME, general medical expenses. If there are any deans of medical schools who would like to help me restructure the GME and indirect medical costs in order to get more primary-care physicians produced in this country, we would certainly change the incentives.

There was a reference made to the very large administrative costs in our present system. Dr. Foote responded: "It is true that we have tremendous administrative overhead; however, some of the HMOs have administrative costs below those of Canada, so a single-payer system is not necessarily the only way to cut administrative costs, but it is one way. The fact that Americans like choice tends to some extent to drive costs up. Choice has a cost."

Reference

1. S. Bartlett Foote, *Managing the Medical Arms Race: Innovation and Public Policy in the Medical Device Industry* (Berkeley: University of California Press, 1992).

PART II

•

ECONOMICS AND MANAGEMENT

CHAPTER 6

Health Care Economics: Today and Tomorrow

WILLIAM PIERSKALLA
University of California at Los Angeles
and
MARTHA BRIZENDINE JENKINSON
Wharton School
University of Pennsylvania

"What changed in 1992?...It is *now* a middle-class issue.... There are a whole set of issues which are bringing fear to the entire middle class."

"The specialists are really the endangered species here.... Our medical schools turn out about four specialists to every primary-care doctor—this behavior will change."

"We almost never put in labor-saving technologies today—rather, we utilize labor-consuming technologies."

"There will be an emphasis on prevention, cost reduction, and continuous quality improvement."

Health care expenditures per capita in the United States are considerably higher than the GNP of some of our major trading partners and competitor nations. We spend about $2,000 per person in the U.S. for health care, whereas our nearest competitors are more in the range of $600 to $1,200 per person. Britain has capped its health expenditures, and has done so for a long time, utilizing global budgets. Germany has had an extensive rise in its health care costs, around 5 percent per year compounded in real terms until it presently capped its budget at about 9 percent. Japan's costs are starting to get a little out of hand. That nation has a large aging population, and it has not capped its expenditures in the same way that the EC countries have.

There are about 40 million uninsured people in the United States. The actual number fluctuates based on unemployment and other factors, but it has been fairly steady for ten years or so. Health insurance costs for employers who pay for health insurance is running around $4,000 per employee per year, a figure projected to rise next year to about $4,400. This is a doubling over the past five years, and it is the basis of the problem we are facing. Business costs for health care are up again in 1993 by about 10 to 12 percent, with 3 percent of that due to inflation—that means a rise of about 7 to 9 percent in real terms. The increase is lower for managed care—about 4 percent—but is higher for indemnity plans.

Why is this a hot topic today? What changed in 1992? We have had this cost crisis for years, and we have had major problems with access to health care for years. It is hot because it is *now* a middle-class issue. It is also a budgetary *deficit* issue. The primary factor is that the middle class in the U.S. is afraid of health care expenditures and the loss of health insurance. They have never been motivated by the idea of what percentage of GNP it is. They *are* motivated by these personal questions:

- "How much does *my* health insurance cost?"
- "How much are *my* cash take-home wages?"
- "How much of *my* cash wages do I have to spend on co-insurance and deductibles?"
- "What if I lose *my* job?"

There also are the issues of exclusion for preexisting conditions. Often employers do not offer insurance because they are in smaller service industries. There are a whole set of issues which are bringing fear to the entire middle class.

What are the factors that affect health care costs? If we consider the annual rates of change in real terms over the past three decades, we find that population factors account for about 1.2 percent of the increase in health care costs. This is due to the growth in population and the aging of the population—factors that relate to demographics. Another much larger factor is economy-wide inflation. A third, but smaller, factor is excessive medical-care costs.

Other factors also represent a relatively large amount. There is a major distinction that is critical to this analysis, and that is the *growth* in costs. We are not referring to the $800 to $900 billion, but rather to the growth that is added on each year. Since 1970 costs have increased from about 8 percent to about 14 percent of the GNP. In real terms the growth rate has been averaging 5 to 6 percent per year, with very little change after adjusting for inflation. The major factors affecting health care costs are:

- demographics
- input prices
- volume and intensity
- waste

One interesting component to the *demographics* is the growth of centenarians in the U.S.—from a little over 10,000 in 1960 to an estimated 100,000 in the year 2000 to a projected 1,000,000 in the year 2050! *Input prices* are the costs of inputs that go into health care in the form of wages and supplies. *Volume and intensity* is the area that concerns us in this setting—it is a catch-all for such factors as big technology (machines, equipment, special facilities, operating rooms, etc.), as well as small technologies (small instruments and new lab tests, for example). It includes the use of older technologies for new purposes, such as diagnostics, imaging, laboratory uses, etc. Also included in the volume and intensity category are some elements of defensive medicine—the additional things we do that wouldn't be done if we could look a little differently at the liability issues involved. Volume and intensity also includes more specialty care (a form of technology)—we pay specialists more than we pay primary-care providers. The cost of excess capacity is also included. We have about a third of our hospital beds unoccupied at any given time. There is also a lot of other excess capacity in ancillary and supportive services.

The last major factor is *waste,* which includes administrative complexity, difficulties in billing, and diseconomies of scope—the fact that we have so many different products and activities in the same institution that there is often a costly level of congestion and confusion as well as costly billing and payment mechanisms. There are also small area variations in costs which affect the overall levels of costs but not their rates of growth. For example, why do we use so many more resources in one area than in another area? There are also the issues of the tax laws favoring employees, at least the employees who buy health care, because health care is paid *before* tax deduction and there is little incentive for patients to limit their utilization of the health care system. Then there are the standard issues of greed and fraud which also come into play.

Consider the differences between the growth in costs and the base of costs. As certain elements of the cost structure in health care have changed, the overall annual growth rate of 5 to 6 percent continues unabated. This growth factor is the push, the driving force, for our concerns and problems. A major shift in the base, for example, resulted from DRGs changing from retrospective payments to prospective payments; that cut our costs for a *short* period of time. But the growth trend continued. The same thing happened with the introduction of HMOs—although it cut costs, it didn't affect long-term growth trends. We can save money in the short terms by cutting costs via uniform billing, test reform, etc., but for the long-term impact we have to look at the fundamental growth trends.

Minnesota's health care costs are about 15 percent below the national average. Minnesotans don't pay as much as we do. But this year employers in Minnesota are anticipating a 12 to 15 percent rise in their expenditures from the lower base. They haven't changed the trend. Many things being proposed that will result in shifts in the base are unlikely to change that fundamental trend of 5 to 6 percent growth, annually compounded.

As mentioned above, about 1.2 percent of cost *growth* is due to demographics—population and aging. We cannot control those— they are part of the system we live in. About 2 percent is input prices. We can exert control there—on physician wages, supplies, nurses' wages, for example. The rest is volume and intensity—2 to 3 percent. This is where technology is the major driver.

There are a number of different proposals to change the health care system. The *employer mandate plan* is where all employers must furnish a basic package to their employees regardless of company size. There is usually a pay or play clause—if your rates are too high you may get a tax credit or voucher—and thus small businesses will be helped. There are mechanisms proposed for a large employer to opt out and pay into a government plan via a standard payroll tax of about 7 percent to 9 percent. There are really no cost controls in that approach.

Another proposal is *managed competition*, utilizing HIPCs (health insurance purchasing cooperatives), more recently called Health Alliances, to approve and monitor qualified plans. These are large cooperatives of employers (possibly including the government) and other groups, who invest in health care for their employees. Large purchasers can wield clout in the market regarding costs and quality. In some cases, these groups also purchase the coverage. The idea behind the managed competition or HIPC approach is that HIPCs will act as informed, cost-conscious surrogates for consumers in granting qualification and approval to plans. This addresses the problem of most consumers not knowing how to buy health care intelligently. It is not like buying an automobile or personal computer; it is a very difficult purchase decision, and most people don't have the necessary knowledge or information. The HIPCs will provide that for us as a surrogate. An additional part of the managed competition proposal is that the employer's contribution and the tax exclusion will be limited to the lowest cost plan, which will encourage providers to develop low costs in order to get the business.

Another aspect is payer-rate regulation, to limit the rates paid by private payers as well as those paid by Medicare and Medicaid. There could be some differences allowed, but by and large the idea is to make the payment amounts the same for every payer, which will avoid cost shifting. As the proposal now stands, there may not be limits on volume. It is amazing how the health care system can create demand. What happens if you try to control costs this way is that there is the creation of demand and increased volume—and costs actually go up.

The major cost-control proposal being discussed is *global budgets*. There are two types of global budgets being discussed—one caps only the public budget; the other caps the total budget. Not many people are thinking in terms of only the public budget; there is usually some combination with private budgets. For example, assume that we set total spending at no more than 14 percent of the GDP. You could also limit spending by sector, such as by providers. You can put limits on capitation rates or on the amount of insurance per head that will be paid on an annual basis. Or you can put limits on price to providers—that is price control.

The global budgets in many EC countries include capitation limits and an annually negotiated fee schedule with physicians and other providers. They also annually negotiate budgets for hospitals or use a DRG-type point system, and they have strictly limited access to capital. Capital access is determined by some global budget administrative authority. That administrative authority is known by different names in each country but is essentially a national health board. In the U.S. a National Health Board is also being considered. It would be another big, new regulatory agency that would approve new technologies using cost-effectiveness studies and outcomes research, and it would help set medical practice guidelines.

What might be in the Clinton proposal? Perhaps the following components:

- Global Budget or Price Controls,
- Managed Competition,
- Managed Care,
- Universal Coverage,
- Employer Mandates,
- A National Health Board.

Managed care means a greater emphasis on primary care and much more limited direct access to specialists. There would be universal coverage, probably phased in because the costs could be substantial—perhaps $50 to $150 billion. It would likely include employer mandates, because employer payment is already an integral part of the system and we cannot change it very easily. It could also streamline billing processes, constrain drug prices, probably reform the malpractice laws, go to a community rating instead of an individual rating for diseases and insurance payments, call for more prevention and primary care, and probably do more in the AIDS treatment area.

HIPC and provider health-delivery plans could have the following changes and factors:

- Managed Competition, through bidding and contracting;
- Managed Care, through primary-care gatekeepers;
- All Payer Rate Regulation/Community Rating of risk;
- Tort Reform, either directly by law or indirectly by clinical pathways;
- Drug Regulation of prices through large bulk purchasing;
- Simplified Billing to all payers;
- Global Budgets via annual capitation fees.

What would this mean to the management and structure of the health care industry and what might it mean to the R&D community? Consider managed competition and managed care—the HIPCs will probably have the following kind of impact on the delivery of care or on provider processes:

- increased primary-care alternatives,
- decreased costs in the short term,
- increase in process and outcomes quality,
- decreased breadth of physician decision making,
- reduced number and income of specialties,
- reduced number of acute beds and bed-days used,
- increase in mergers and alliances,
- more competition on price and quality.

There will probably be increased primary-care alternatives—there will be more and more shifts to HMO-types of activity for most people who have paid insurance, whether or not it is paid by private employers. There will be increased use of facilities outside of the hospital (home health care, for example). There will probably be some decreased health care costs in the short term—perhaps quite significant reductions. There will be an increase in the use of process and outcomes quality information in making decisions about health care and about which institutions and which providers one would go to. There will be reduced breadth of physician decision making—more clinical protocols or clinical pathways will be written in order to reduce the variation in treatment and practice patterns, and also to reduce the resources being used to treat particular problems. There will be a reduced number and income of specialists.

The current levels and future output of specialists will be greatly affected. Specialists are really the endangered species here. About one-third of our physicians are primary-care physicians; two-thirds are specialists of various types. We have the lowest number of primary-care physicians in the developed industrialized world. Other countries have numbers much higher. In Britain 70 percent of all physicians are primary-care providers. Specialists in most of the rest of the world only get cases from the primary-care doctors. As we move more to HPICs this will also be true here. Our medical schools turn out about four specialists to every primary-care doctor; this behavior will change, and incentives are already being structured to accomplish that. We might see some specialists going back to primary-care practice in order to get enough business and a sufficient income.

There will be a reduced number of acute beds and bed-days used. We already have an excess capacity of about 33 percent. Some hospitals will be closed down; others will merge or will be used for longer-term care or different activities. There will be major increases in mergers, alliances, and joint ventures.

Minnesota is already experimenting with this particular aspect of health care reform. There are fourteen firms in Minnesota which got together to form a HIPC. They are firms whose employees use about $200 million worth of care per year, and who constitute about 6 percent of the market there. RFPs were issued to various health providers. A major coalition involving two HMOs, the Mayo Clinic, and a large group practice presented a bid for that care against Blue Cross, Blue Shield, and others. The first group was the low bidder and was awarded the business. Other hospitals and groups are realizing they now have to form coalitions. There is an ever greater demand for primary-care physicians and a decreasing demand for specialists in those coalitions. We will see more of these mergers and relationships in the management area. The providers in turn will try to build their power to countervail the power of the HIPCs.

What does this mean for technology? Such major coalitions and mergers means that the resulting entities are not going to buy as much technology and they are going to use their technology more effectively. Instead of having 300 to 400 percent excess capacity in some of their technology areas, over time they are going to reduce it to 150 percent or less of needed capacity. This will be true of beds and in all other technologies. We will see more competition on price and quality.

Making global budgets is a strategy that actually decreases the 6 percent growth rate, because it puts a cap on total spending. In a global-budget environment we can expect:

- price and quality competition/market niches,
- a slow diffusion of cost-increasing technology,
- an increase in labor-saving technologies,
- an increase in salaried physicians,
- an emphasis on prevention,
- a reduction in system capacities,
- a reduction in speed of access,

- a strong emphasis on cost reduction and continuous quality improvement (CQI).

We almost never institute labor-saving technologies today—rather, we utilize labor-consuming technologies. In the future, there will be an emphasis on prevention, cost reduction, and continuous quality improvement.

The trends in research funding are likely to be:

- basic research funding will decrease (not so much from government sources as from private industry, which will not see the same growth markets for new technology as at present)
- more cost-effectiveness criteria for developmental research and more governmental approaches before the introduction of new technologies
- less overall funding for developmental research
- a shift of R&D to *true* cost-saving technologies

There will be a shift in R&D to *true* cost-saving technologies—most of the past and present cost analysis is individual- or item-specific and does not look at the system as a whole. In fact, even though it may look like you save some cost on an individual basis, when you look at the total system, almost all new technologies and new health care–delivery approaches usually add more people, more facilities, processes, etc. When we think of cost analysis, we have to think of it as a system analysis and not just as an individual technology or individual item analysis. That is a very critical point.

What is likely to happen in the short term is difficult to say. There are 741 registered health lobbyists in Washington, D.C. Remember what happened to catastrophic coverage for Medicare when it went through—everybody wanted it until they had to pay for it. That caused a major uproar and the bill was rescinded rather rapidly. Also, nobody is really talking about long-term care, which is a big cost-driver and will increase. Long-term care for the United States? I don't know what it will be. In those countries with public long-term care financing, the aging of their population is leading to a great financial burden on the working population.

The European community seems to have some grip on most of the problems: universal coverage, cost control, and controlled access. They have universal budget caps, decentralized purchasing agencies to buy health services for customers, and growing competition among both public and private providers. There is quality self-regulation in most of their systems. There are capitation payments to primary-care providers, who are the gatekeepers to the system. They have far fewer specialists and they have both capped and separate capital budgets. Although each individual system has unique features and its own set of problems, almost all of the European systems are converting to such a model. We are also moving in that direction.

CHAPTER 7

Discussion: Continuous Quality Improvement

SUSAN HORN
Intermountain Health Care (IHC)
Salt Lake City, Utah

"The best way to decrease health care costs is to improve quality."

"Randomized control trials...would be too restrictive...because we are looking at *all* aspects of care."

"We are controlling costs by finding out what works and what doesn't."

"We must find better ways to make health information more accessible to people who are trying to find the best medical practice."

The best way to decrease health care costs is to improve quality. Our goal at IHC has been to find the best outcomes of care for the least necessary cost. We have been structuring our health care system so that we can find and use effective, efficient processes across the continuum of care. We don't just look at what is happening with inpatient settings; we also look at the ambulatory setting. We never look at winning in just one sector; we look at the total picture to find the best outcomes for the least necessary cost over the whole spectrum of health care expenditures. We have to document optimal outcomes and routinely generate scientifically valid clinical knowledge in the course of delivering care, in order that we can continually improve quality, cost, and the processes, as well as demonstrate that we have the most effective, efficient care.

How do we do it? There has been much resistance in the medical community to moving in this direction. We had similar experiences to those shared by Kilpatrick (Chapter 9)—the system really did not want to change. We have been able to convince medical people in the Salt Lake region and across the nation and the world (many of whom have come to learn how we are doing this in Salt Lake City) to take the gold standard that we were using before—randomized control trials—and put it in a new framework, which we are calling *clinical practice improvement*, a branch of continuous quality improvement, and then find out what works best. We select areas we want to study the same as we would for a randomized trial. We use a clinical-quality monitor to collect the data, just as physicians or other providers would collect it on their charts. It is not a separate data-collection effort. Then we go on to make improvements in the process of care based on those facts.

As Samuel Thier indicated in Chapter 1, we must have a basis in fact, not solely on opinion. In terms of the clinical-quality monitors, we feel that every patient who comes into the hospital with a particular problem should become part of an effort to find the best care. We look at severity of illness, differences, and indicators for treatment, so everybody coming in can become part of the effort to find the best process of care.

How do we find those best processes? In randomized control trials we have to explicitly specify everything ahead of time. Here that would be too restrictive, because we are looking at *all* aspects of care. We are not just looking at the big, new technologies. We look at little things, such as when is the most appropriate time to deliver a prophylactic antibiotic before surgery, how to prevent adverse drug events, or how to prevent pressure sores from developing. These are all things that are not big items when you look at them in terms of new technologies, but they end up costing a great deal in terms of health care. We determine the best processes by three methods. One is to measure how people are being treated, feed this information back to practitioners, and have them converge to the pattern that appears to be giving the best outcome for the least necessary cost. Feedback of data does cause change to happen.

A second methodology, when it is appropriate, is that we get experts together and ask them to develop very precise protocols. That means that for every physiological problem, we decide, as a team, what to do. That again is often a difficult process. As it begins to come together and as physicians begin to think in that direction, however, it can have enormous benefits in terms of decreased costs. Finally, and this is becoming more prevalent now, we take external sets of process specifications, apply them internally, and then modify and improve them over time. These are, in essence, the steps we take to utilize a randomized control trial format to find the best outcomes for the least necessary cost.

Where does this lead in terms of the bottom line? One example is represented by data for DRG 209, Total Hip. Ten IHC hospitals perform this procedure; in the rest of Utah there are also ten non-IHC hospitals that perform it. Using the rest of Utah as the basis, IHC's length of stay in total is about 23.6 percent below the rest of Utah; it is 23.9 percent below in terms of average cost and 23.3 percent below in terms of average charges. Every IHC facility has used a clinical practice improvement model to look at how they are treating this DRG. They were directed to do this by IHC corporate policy. The global ramifications are evident. There are some non-IHC hospitals that also have costs below the other non-IHC institutions, but overall every IHC institution has achieved significant cost savings—and this was only the first step. Now we are beginning to pool our processes together to see if we can find the most optimal.

The data for coronary artery bypass surgery (DRG 106 and 107) offers another example. In this case there are only three IHC facilities and three non-IHC facilities in the state that perform this procedure. One IHC hospital has a smaller sample size; it has not yet initiated a clinical practice improvement effort. It is more like the non-IHC hospitals in terms of cost. Two other IHC hospitals put in a major effort in this area, with great effects in terms of improving the quality of care. That is the kind of evidence we are able to share with practitioners to point out to them that if they participate with us in this endeavor, they will end up being able to show to health care payers that they are delivering the best quality of care for the least necessary cost.

The overall effect of this endeavor can be seen when we compare hospitals in Utah to those in the rest of the nation. My analysis has been adjusted for case mix, wages, teaching, and the other things in the Health Care Financing Administration model. Charge differentials and cost differentials were examined. Since 1987 Utah, and IHC in particular, have been below the rest of the nation in terms of charges. Many people attribute such results to the basic life-style in Utah. IHC has always been lower than non-IHC hospitals with regard to charges. However, as the years progressed to 1991, IHC became ever more efficient, with now a 43.2 percent lower charge than the rest of the nation, whereas non-IHC is nearer to the rest of the nation and in 1991 was only 10.7 percent below the national average. However, the real bottom line refers to cost. In 1987 and 1988 the costs at IHC were slightly (2 percent) higher than at the non-IHC hospitals in the state of Utah. They were still below the national average, but IHC did not have an advantage. In 1988 clinical practice improvement studies began. In 1988–89 we were 2 percent better than non-IHC. In 1990 it was 4 percent and in 1991 it was 10 percent better than the rest of Utah and 22.8 percent below the national average. For 1992 the IHC figures were about 16 percent below the rest of Utah. The direction is right. We are controlling costs by finding out what works and what doesn't.

About 500 clinical-practice improvement studies have already been conducted at IHC, but that is only the tip of the iceberg. There are still hundreds and hundreds of processes that we need to study to find out what works best and how we can get the best outcomes for the least necessary cost. We believe that efforts in this direction are one very important aspect in the control of health care costs. It turns out that foreign nations—Spain and England, for example— are beginning to turn to Clinical Practice Improvement (CPI); they feel that price controls alone no longer will be able to solve health care cost problems. We have to find out what works and what does not work.

The fact that we have a computerized medical record system at IHC means that we can look at many items of information about a patient, such as details as to how severely ill the patient is, and relate that to the process of care. The fact that that data is easily accessible is what has helped us to move as quickly as we have in finding the best medical practice. We must find better ways to make health information more accessible to people who are trying to find the best medical practice.

CHAPTER 8

Discussion: Health Care Economics and Management

KERRY KILPATRICK
Center for Health Policy and
Management
University of North Carolina
and
ROBERT HUEFNER
Department of Political Science
University of Utah

"We have no mechanisms for making cost-effectiveness trade-offs."

"They spend millions on marketing but very little on productivity improvement."

"Real cost constraints will require more global budgeting or eventually a single-payer system."

Systems engineering is one branch of engineering that relates to the health care cost-containment problem. Also called operations research, management science, or management engineering, it is the branch of engineering that deals exclusively with productivity enhancement. Working in the health care setting is an extraordinarily frustrating experience for systems engineers. Twenty or so years ago when bright-eyed systems engineers tried to make changes in the health care system, we found that the system did not want to change very rapidly. Now things are even worse. How many major teaching hospitals have major industrial engineering operations, as compared to their operations in marketing and planning? They spend millions on marketing but very little on productivity improvement. The frustration is that price times quantity equals expenditures, as Pierskalla (Chapter 6) pointed out; but price times quantity also equals revenues. Somebody's revenues are being reduced as you try to reduce either component of the price times quantity equation.

Reducing costs reduces income for physicians, nurses, and other people in the system. Without the growth in jobs in the health care sector, there wouldn't have been any growth in jobs in this country in the last five years. In some cities, the health care industry is the only industry supporting the economy. In Durham, North Carolina, for example, we no longer call Durham the "City of Tobacco"; it is now the "City of Medicine." The Duke University Medical Center can be thought of as a giant funnel for community resources and for support of the economy.

Can anything be done to save the productivity-enhancing attributes of technology while we are trying to control the cost increases? Pierskalla has suggested global budgeting as one thing that could be done. What is its effect on technology? The stock market has told us that even hints of global budgeting lead the stock market to go downhill. We don't actually assess the trade-offs between what we should be doing, but rather we assess whether this emerging technology is more cost effective than a technology we already have in place.

One fundamental issue is that we spend about a third of our Medicare dollars—roughly 60 billion dollars—on the last year of life. Should those dollars be spent on prenatal care and vaccinations? Should they be spent in other sectors of the economy? We have no mechanisms for making cost-effectiveness trade-offs. Even further down the line, we don't have any mechanism for trading off those dollars with expenditures in education, housing, or infrastructure which might tend over the long-term to alleviate the problems. At one time we thought the 1983 DRG changes were on to something, and then somebody discovered the charge shift, so you could just shift your charges to the other payers. As long as that safety valve is there, we will not have cost constraints. Real cost constraints will require more global budgeting or eventually a single-payer system.

Part of the problem is our inability to do the technological forecasting required to evaluate emerging technologies. Many grant proposals to evaluate emerging technologies are reviewed as inadequate because they do not show sufficient historic data upon which to base the evaluation. That is the point. In order to evaluate emerging technology you have to do some forecasting. We need to be more innovative and put more intellectual capital into technological forecasting for emerging technologies. We need to ask what will happen *if* this technology is successful; what happens if it grows to a certain state; what happens if at a certain point on the learning curve, either in terms of cost or productivity, it is a reasonable technology to adopt. We can do some pretty good technological forecasting, but such evaluation is not being done in the United States although there is some such activity in Europe.

CHAPTER 9

Romance and Realism: The Strategic Vision of the National Institutes of Health

BERNADINE HEALY, M.D.

"Accountability must apply to everyone, whether one looks at biomedical research from the grass roots up or from the top down."

"This puts an obligation on us, each in our own way, to tell the public what we are doing and how it is done. Keep in mind, after all, that the public perception of what we do is not always exact—and when that condition exists, it is our problem."

"Keep listening to the public, and keep talking with them about what we are doing, about the outcomes we are hoping for, about the costs and—by far the most urgent—about the *benefits* that they and their children will see from all we spend and do."

"We must be adaptable,...especially in recognizing critical areas of fundamental research—and then in funding them."

There is an old song they used to sing around closing time in bars —at least that's what I've been told. I'm not going to sing it, because it has about twenty-seven verses and, besides, it's not closing time yet. But the song tells a story about a man who just got married and has come home with his new bride. But when they get home, the woman of his dreams takes out her glass eye, removes her false hair, drops her teeth in a glass, and unstraps her limb prosthesis. By the time she's through, there's not much left. Perhaps most interesting, the title of this song—and the refrain sung after every verse—is "He's a Very Unfortunate Man."

Far be it for the Director of the NIH, who happens to be a woman and who takes great pride in our Women's Health Initiative, to see even a trace of sexism in this old bar song. If *he* is unfortunate, what about *her*? But of course, the "unfortunate" husband was a romantic, expecting the woman of his dreams to be perfect, and was reduced to despair when his romanticism got run over by the freight train of reality.

We know that in the fields of medicine and biology and biomedical engineering there has to be a dose of romanticism—a belief that our heroic efforts and determination can conquer any disease or disability. But something else has to come first—and that is an even larger dose of realism, an acceptance of the facts.

Creating Our Own Future

The unfortunate man's unfortunate wife's glass eye and the rest may be pretty crude stuff compared to an artificial vein engineered from tissue, but both of them deal with reality: we're not perfect, we need help. To consider human disability "unfortunate" is just about as useless as making fun of it: both postures ignore the plain reality that we can do something about human need and imperfection if, instead of wringing our hands over scarce resources, we put our hands to work in the real world. Let's be realists first and then romantics.

The mission statement of the NIH both defines and conditions the essential realism of our strategy: "Science in the pursuit of knowledge to improve human health." This means that ideas and results—especially results—come first. This also means that the real and applicable fruits of scientific work, even when driven by romantic enthusiasm, are more critical than *any* of us as individual scientists and researchers. To be the best, we must have the inspiration and creativity of individual scientists. Therefore the NIH embraces investigator-initiated research by its scientists. But we must at the same time look at national needs.

The importance of assessing public need is at the heart of strategic planning for science. Congressman George Brown, who heads the House Committee on Science, Space, and Technology, recently asked what kinds of research offer the greatest hope and prospect of improving human life. He addressed the question in the context of long-range planning and priority settings. Our NIH Strategic Plan, completed after more than two years of work, carries the title *"Investment* for Humanity." When you manage an investment, you may be looking toward payoffs in the future, but you are accountable to the investors—in our case, the American taxpayers—*every single day in the present.*

This sense of accountability must apply to everyone, whether one looks at biomedical research from the grass roots up or from the top down. My own sense is that it would do all of us a lot of good to take the time—and find the patience—to work through at least one of the congressional authorization or appropriation bills. You will see incredibly detailed congressional top down management. NIH strategic planning has for the first time given us the chance as a scientific community to participate in the process as well.

The next time someone asks you, "What has science done for me lately?" you will see what a strategic question it is. You may do well by pointing to the increases in cancer survival rates or the decreases in deaths from stroke or by describing a new treatment for cystic fibrosis or new drugs for orphan diseases. This is certainly more dramatic and persuasive than telling them about the number of RO1 grants. But you will do even better in answering that question if, in addition to enumerating breakthroughs in extending healthy life or counting the dollars spent in the last fiscal year, you can also describe how our present efforts are directly connected to a better future. And that is the function of the Strategic Plan—that is why we have it and why it belongs to the American Institute for Medical and Biological Engineering as much as it belongs to the National Institutes of Health or to researchers anywhere else. Approach the Plan with a sense of proprietorship, since many of you participated in its development.

The Flexibility of the Plan

The Strategic Plan is, in fact, a vision. It is printed on paper, not chiseled deeply in granite: it is a map for us to use for the time being, for our foreseeable future, not a companion piece to Mount Rushmore. Let me explain with an example or two.

Forty years ago, the Nobel Prize for Medicine was shared by Hans Krebs and Fritz Lipmann for their work on metabolism—particularly for identifying the mechanisms in living organisms for breaking down food molecules to produce adenosine triphosphate (ATP). Considering that the energy released by ATP drives the biological processes needed to sustain life, growth, movement, and reproduction in plants and animals, we can agree that Krebs and Lipmann had taken on one of the burning questions of the day and answered it. But, by an irony we all recognize and understand, their breakthrough removed their work, *as a process*, from the leading edge of science and transferred it, *as an accomplishment*, to the category of received knowledge.

As a second example, take AIDS. Had we written a Strategic Plan or even just a fiscal-year budget about a dozen years ago, AIDS research would have been absent. And for good reason: we didn't know about it. Just as the discovery of the Krebs Cycle put an end to one kind of effort, so the eruption of AIDS has obliged us to begin another. In other words, we have learned that either the great breakthrough or the new calamity are both likely and that any plan must be adaptable.

We must be adaptable, as well, especially in recognizing critical areas of fundamental research and then in funding them. As we identify critical needs—and not only because of a scourge like AIDS but also because of new knowledge we can apply—those areas must be permitted to grow at a different rate than other areas in the national health and research budget. Let me summarize: the Strategic Plan must be flexible enough to respond to changes in the requirements of science and in the needs of the society. And it is.

Perhaps most important of all, the Strategic Plan will increase our flexibility. A plan like this is not intended to control or influence any individual investigator's pursuit of discovery, but, on the contrary, to influence and, as far as possible, condition the *environment* in which biomedical researchers operate—and operate freely, as creative individuals.

Planning is really no more or less than the dose of realism, and the Strategic Plan's six trans-NIH objectives are fully responsive to the real changes in both science and society. Think of it in terms of a family.

1. Critical Science and Technology

There are no stepchildren here. However, the needs of one child may lead it to cry out louder at times—and for good reason. That is happening in the family of biomedical research today; so our first objective is to ensure that we treat critical areas of science and technology in basic biology as priorities all across the NIH. The critical areas we have identified are molecular medicine, immunology and vaccines, structural biology, cellular and integrative biology, and, of course, biotechnology and bioengineering.

These critical areas of science and technology are providing today—and will be providing in the foreseeable future—the new and dynamic fundamental knowledge on which virtually all NIH activities must rely. As a matter of plain fact and good practice, the several disciplines mentioned in the first objective will be relying on one another. For example, the efforts of integrative biologists to further our understanding of the human brain are likely to give us fundamental information necessary for the development of new preventive, therapeutic, and restorative measures which might alleviate, remedy, or even reverse the effects of central-nervous-system disabilities. As their understanding of the life of the human cell and, especially, of specific cellular functions advances, the use of cells as therapeutic agents will be shifting from concept to technique. And while the concept may serve the bioengineer as the romantic jolt to begin a new investigation, it will be the possibility of a technique, the product of basic science, that will provide us with the realistic environment for getting down to work and solving the problem.

In truth, we will be solving more than one problem. The first and obvious one is the problem of improving human health. The second problem takes us into the heart of the American economy. The business pages of the newspapers are still debating the relative merits of a manufacturing economy as opposed to a service economy—and perhaps they will forever and we may never be any the wiser for all the quarrels on this subject. But no one is arguing the importance of advancing technology, whether applied by manufacturing or as a service to other industries. Both historical fact and future necessity prove that truth.

As Americans, we have both the tradition and the patents to point to as evidence of our preeminence in invention and technology. The MIT economist Lester Thurow recently has argued eloquently that technology, in all its varieties as an "industry," is the first among equals of all the key industries that will enable America to compete head to head with Europe and Japan.

2. Critical Health Needs

This is the point to which we must *always* return, because applying critical science and technology to improve the health of the American people will shape and control any strategy we may agree on. The individual NIH institutes—each focusing on specific diseases or questions of human health—are the tactical agents for realizing the NIH's overall strategy. If they are going to succeed, then we must accomplish our second objective, which is to strengthen the ability of the nation's biomedical research enterprise to respond to current and emerging public health needs.

Some of these critical health needs are basic environmental biology, health and human behavior, disease control and prevention, the health of women and of underserved minority populations, and aging. Biomedical engineering has a major role to play in virtually all of these critical health needs.

3. Intellectual Capital

The third trans-NIH objective—the renewal and growth of intellectual capital—is critical to the first two. Winston Churchill said, "The empires of the future are the empires of the mind." He spoke those words fifty years ago—and *we* are the future he was talking about. The spice trade or oil wells or even high technology will not invariably enrich us or give us power—only ideas will. We can put our greatest faith in products of the mind. We can only be as creative and successful, therefore, as the scientists who make up our enterprises. To this end, our strategy depends on our efforts to encourage and foster the present and the future creative arenas of the men and women who are carrying on biomedical and behavioral research.

We can accomplish some of this with training and career development and by deliberately seeking out a talent base that is both robust and diverse. But again, we need a dose of realism. Promising young people are shying away from biomedical research, and the reason isn't romantic—it's money. Talented U.S. post-docs are becoming harder and harder to find, and trained researchers are turning to other fields. This may be the biggest threat from lean NIH budgets: young people see no future and turn away. We must do better in career development or find ourselves fresh out of the intellectual capital we need to invest in our future. We have come up with some mechanisms, like the Shannon Award and Junior R01 grants, to try and address the need to attract and retain young scientists. But we need more.

4. Research Capacity

Our fourth objective—one closely related to the development of human capital—is to attend to the needs for research resources, instrumentation, lab facilities, and enabling technologies like computers and software in order to give physical, and applicable, expression to the ideas and discoveries of biomedical research.

5. Stewardship of Public Resources

This objective, of course, means spending a lot of money—$10 billion currently—that belongs to the taxpayers. It means that we must be efficient and responsible, honest and fair, and that we must let the public know what is happening with their money. Their investment will only last as long as their confidence in us.

And this puts an obligation on us, each in our own way, to tell the public what we are doing and how it is done. Keep in mind, after all, that the public perception of what we do is not always exact—and when that condition exists, it is our problem. For example, I recently heard someone who is pretty knowledgeable about medical affairs refer to bioengineers as "divine tinkerers, but on a grand scale." For him, "on a grand scale" was the operative phrase, but maybe it was not for the public.

There is still a romantic notion that all great research is still stuck in the nineteenth century—that devices or techniques that may, for example, enable a deaf person to perceive sound will be "invented" by an inspired individual noodling around at a bench covered with spare parts and about ten dollars' worth of stuff from the hardware store. It's an image of the romantic hero colored with a little looniness—you know, Alexander Graham Bell meets Gyro

Gearloose, with a touch of Archimedes jumping out of his bathtub and running through the streets shouting "Eureka!"

We are looking to three-dimensional imaging that will enable surgeons to perform laparoscopic suturing and knot tying as easily as in open surgery. We are looking to extracorporeal livers, capable of purifying a patient's serum for a few days or weeks while waiting for a transplant. And we are looking to the technology and the therapeutic benefit that we would achieve from biohybrid artificial organs—pancreas, lymph node, nerve, and muscle—in the treatment of various diseases. You know our progress has been produced by cooperation and interdisciplinary labor, not by the lone genius; and you know that ten dollars won't buy the biomedical devices, the processing technologies, or the biomaterials to get the job done.

6. Earning the Public's Trust

Divine tinkering, indeed—*and* on a grand scale of both human and financial resources. It is the grand scale—why the scale must be so grand to produce such grand results—that we must never forget to *explain* to the men and women of America. For we will fail to convince the public of our good stewardship if we do not make sure that we are earning their trust, our sixth objective. In part, this requires us to hold the NIH to the highest standards. In part, this requires us to respond to the social, legal, and ethical issues that health research must inevitably raise. And in part, it requires us to keep listening to the public and to keep talking with them about what we are doing, about the outcomes we are hoping for, about the costs and—by far the most urgent—about the *benefits* that they and their children will see from all we spend and do.

This tells you the obvious: that all six of these objectives are connected. For example, you cannot really separate the building of a scientific infrastructure from research capacity or separate the promotion of critical science and technology from the formation of intellectual capital. So everything the NIH does or finances must ultimately and clearly connect with the health of Americans.

The Strategic Plan will provide a blueprint of our biomedical research enterprise, describing what it takes for us to succeed and to achieve the high expectations the public has for medical research. The Strategic Plan connects our romantic strivings to our sense of reality by letting us keep our eyes on the stars while we keep our feet on the ground.

Discussion

With Ms. Healy's announced resignation as Director of the NIH, there was concern as to who will champion her strategic vision and implement the Strategic Plan. It was noted that neither the president nor the Office of Science and Technology Policy necessarily support the NIH Strategic Plan, but that the Plan's recommendations are being seriously considered.

Another discussant noted that there is general agreement in the research community on many aspects of the plan and that "most of the pieces have the broad support of the community, make a lot of sense, and should move forward."

It was noted that the bioengineering community feels "very positive about the process. It was the first time there has been a way for the bioengineering community to enter into such a planning process. We are very pleased that there is a specific focus on biotechnology and bioengineering in the strategic plan."

In response to a comment and a question dealing with research-funding priorities, Dr. Healy said, "You are alluding to a question which you are perhaps too polite to ask. 'Why is biomedical engineering a stepchild in the biomedical research community?' I think this is in part due to the fractionation and hierarchy of disciplines. Disciplinary fractionation does none of us any good. Perhaps the recent silicone breast-implant problem is a good example of intellectual discrimination. Drugs are well evaluated by the NIH and by the regulatory process, but device research and evaluation is not well funded within NIH. Why weren't silicone breast implants studied? Where is the biomedical science base? The biomedical engineering community needs to be more assertive regarding appropriate research needs and resources." She continued this discussion in response to a question on the regulatory process, saying that the silicone breast-implant story is a tragedy of science more than a problem in regulation.

In response to a question regarding congressional micro-management of well-run government agencies, including NIH, Dr. Healy responded that NIH is an extraordinary political football; its authorization bill establishes and requires a variety of committees, bureaucracies, and red tape: "We go through silly exercises that divert our energies and resources from what we should be doing.

NIH gets more micromanagement than most other government agencies because the public is so interested in health and in biomedical research, and we of course want to be and have to be accountable and responsive; but that is no excuse for excessive congressional micromanagement."

In response to a question dealing with behavioral and nutrition studies, Dr. Healy said that these are trans-NIH areas and that a stronger science base is required. "Nothing is more important to health than adequate nutrition. Behavior is a strong thrust throughout NIH. Behavioral studies are an integrated part of biomedical research today, and they could provide a very important role for biomedical engineering. It is exciting that the life sciences appear to be coming together in a number of areas, including the behavioral sciences."

In regard to a comment on training and education, Dr. Healy responded, "No one seems to be planning or developing resources for education." She referred to a study dealing with the number of scientists and engineers per capita: "We led the world many years ago. We have slipped considerably. Japan and Germany have improved their position. These results are a measure of national value and national investment in its own future. Adequate education and training of scientists and engineers has been left out of the dialogue in this country, although it is prominent in the NIH Strategic Plan. The single biggest challenge we face is the development of science and engineering talent for our future."

Editor's Reference

1. *Investment for Humanity: A Strategic Vision for the National Institutes of Health* (Washington, D.C.: National Institute of Health, 1993)—call 301–496–9285 for a copy.

PART III

•

INCENTIVES AND NEW PROGRAMS

•
CHAPTER 10
•

Technologies, Incentives, and Health Care Costs: What Is in Our Future?

BURTON A. WEISBROD
Northwestern University

"Incentives matter, and society sets them—although often unwittingly.... R&D incentives can be changed; technological change does not 'just happen.'"

"We should be...focused on ways to redirect R&D so that tomorrow's health care technology is less costly than today's."

"Advances in knowledge about health care treatment and prevention are not chance events."

"Public policy is now in search of a "basic package" of health care services to be guaranteed to our entire population.... What is "basic" today depends very much on what is possible today, not on what was possible in the past."

"The kinds of new technologies developed in recent decades would have taken very different forms if the incentives facing the R&D sector had been different."

73

"How can public policy go about redirecting health care R&D toward cost-reducing technologies? . . . Establish large prizes for
cost-reducing technologies."

"Society does not have to simply respond to tomorrow's technology; we can shape it."

"What is meant by technology? . . . It is simply knowledge."

Is technology the culprit behind the explosion of health care costs
—or is it a savior? Could it be both? What is the future for health
care technology in an era of cost containment, and is that future
within our control? What is our vision for the kind of health care
technology we seek to develop?

Tomorrow's state of technology depends on today's incentives
in the R&D sector, and public policy can profoundly change those
incentives. This is the case in health care as it is elsewhere in the
economy. Thus, as we work to control health care costs, we must
recognize the profound long-term effects we can have on incentives
for developing new technology. Public policy to control those costs
will also shape incentives to develop new knowledge; in the process, these incentives will determine the state of technology that
our children will inherit.

Sound national policy requires that we understand that soaring
health care expenditures are not the result of increased costs of providing the same service we were providing twenty, thirty, or forty
years ago. Most of today's health care diagnostic and treatment capabilities did not even exist a few decades ago. Spiraling health
care costs are clearly a serious problem, but the problem is not that
we are getting less for our money. Rather, we are paying more and
getting more—we are consuming a steadily improving and expanding set of health services. At the close of World War II we were
spending little or no money at all on intensive-care hospital units,
on artificial hips, knees, and other joints, and on coronary bypass
surgery; they were unknown.

This focus on technological change is directed at the new diagnostic tests, surgical advances, drug therapies, and other advances
that are occurring with dizzying frequency. By emphasizing technology as a driving force, I hope to shift the terms of the policy de-

bate: we should be less preoccupied with solutions that hold a promise of instant gratification in the form of slower growth in prices of particular health care resources—such as prescription drugs and diagnostic equipment—and become more focused on ways to redirect R&D so that tomorrow's health care technology is less costly than today's. We make a mistake if we concentrate only on the costs of health care services that are *now* available; in just a few years there will be a vastly different array of services. What they will be like, and what their costs will be, are not preordained; they are the fundamental questions facing health policy planners.

What is meant by "technology"? It could be hardware, machinery, or equipment, of course; but it need not be. It is simply knowledge—knowledge that is sometimes embodied in equipment and devices such as CT scanners or laser devices for cataract surgery, sometimes embodied in pharmaceuticals and vaccines, and sometimes embodied in people, as, for example, in the knowledge of surgeons about a new surgical technique or of consumers about how to conduct a self-examination for breast or testicular tumors.

Once technology is viewed as knowledge, it becomes easier to see the possibility that public policy can affect incentives for the R&D sector to pursue one form of advance in knowledge rather than another. It then follows that advances in knowledge about health care treatment and prevention are not chance events; they are, in general, results of planned scientific research and related engineering development. The kernel of this theme is that medical R&D is influenced by the anticipated rewards, and these rewards come through the health care finance system. *Incentives matter,* and society sets them—although often unwittingly.

Though my focus is on ways that public policy can alter future health care technology, I am not suggesting that technological forces are the only elements of health care policy. They are not. We are, and should be, interested in the pricing of health care resources. We are, and should be, interested in ending the "job lock" effect of employer-based health care insurance, which prevents workers from moving to more preferable jobs because of fear of losing health care insurance coverage. And, as a civilized society, we are, and should be, searching for a political-social consensus on our obligations to meet the health care needs of the poor.

These are all matters deserving action. Still, as society struggles to establish policy for overall cost containment in health care, the

R&D sector and its incentives cry out for attention. Our goal should be to develop new cost-reducing technologies while we reduce efforts to develop technologies that improve quality of care but increase costs in the process. To do this we should establish incentives for the enormously creative and responsive health care R&D sector to shift its efforts toward cost-reducing technologies. A public policy that favors cost cutting over quality enhancement is a bitter pill; but if we are to succeed in the long-term in reining in health care costs, there is no other option.

R&D incentives can be changed. Technological change does not "just happen"; it is heavily influenced by public policy, although often in unintended ways. It was not inevitable that recent decades would bring forth the kinds of innovations that we now take for granted; a different incentive structure would have brought different results. The dramatic difference between the technological innovations in health care and those in education illustrate the powerful effect of incentives. If schooling were financed the way we have financed health care, each child would receive a battery of diagnostic tests at the beginning of the school year, teachers would then determine what kind of education each child "needed," that education would be provided to the child, the costs of the education would be calculated, and the school would send a bill to a governmental agency or private insurer, which would in turn remit a check. Imagine what that would have meant for the development of educational technology: anything that teachers found to be effective would have a ready and profitable market, whatever the cost! It is no coincidence that today's hospital is vastly different from the typical hospital of 1960, while the fifth-grade classroom of today and that of 1960 are virtually indistinguishable.

In health care, as elsewhere in the economy, higher quality is normally more costly. Sometimes, of course, it has been possible to increase the quality of health services while also cutting costs. The polio vaccine, for example, not only virtually eliminated this devastating disease of youth but also in the process eliminated the high-cost iron-lung technology. Similarly, certain drugs have come to be substituted for high-cost ulcer surgery. Yet most technological advances in recent decades have not been cost-reducing. MRI diagnostic devices, organ transplants, and techniques for keeping babies weighing two pounds (or even less) alive have expanded our health care options but have also increased costs. Rather than substituting for even more costly measures, they have provided additional ways to sustain life or to detect problems that then require costly treatment. These new technologies have much to commend them, but cost reduction is not one of them.

To see the overall effect of technological change over recent decades, ask yourself what the level of health care expenditures would be now if the state of technology had been "frozen" at, for example, its state in 1950. We would be unable to spend money on most of the high-cost techniques that we take for granted today. People with head injuries could not be examined with costly MRI equipment, AIDS victims could not be treated with costly AZT, people with diseased livers could not obtain transplants, and people with kidney disease could not obtain dialysis. Many people would suffer or die prematurely, but health care costs would be lower—in my judgment, far lower.

Public policy can and should set the incentives for health care R&D knowingly and with recognition of their consequences. But we have not done so. To see how some potent incentives have revolutionized health care, let us review some history. By understand-

YEAR

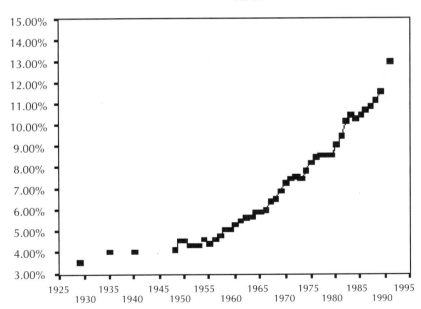

Figure 1. Health Care Expenditures in the U.S., 1929–1991 as a Percentage of the GNP.

Sources: *Statistical Abstract of the United States;* and *Historical Statistics: Colonial Times to 1970,* Part 1, Series B249.

Country	Percent Growth
Iceland	650
Spain	261
Japan	234
Switzerland	233
Norway	227
Netherlands	218
United States	**215**
Belgium	212
Italy	209
France	205
Mean	197
Sweden	191
Finland	190
Ireland	185
Austria	183
Germany	174
Denmark	167
Greece	166
New Zealand	157
United Kingdom	156
Canada	156
Australia	154

Figure 2. Growth of Health Care Expenditures
as a Percentage of the Gross Domestic Product (1960–1987).
Source: Calculated from data in *Health Affairs,* Fall 1989, page 170.

ing how we came to spend one-seventh of our entire national output on health care, we perhaps can see how to change the future. Some historical facts follow.

Fact one. The explosion of health care costs, now at 14 percent of the Gross National Product (GNP), and rising, is relatively recent—a post-World War II phenomenon (see Figure 1). Not generally recognized is that between 1929 (the earliest year for which data is available) and the early 1950s, the share of the GNP devoted to health care barely changed, hovering around 4.0 to 4.5 percent. Since then something new has been happening in health care.

Fact two. Whatever has occurred during this period has been a worldwide phenomenon and not just limited to the United States. Although the absolute level of health care expenditures is highest in this country, it has been rising everywhere. In fact, for most of the period since 1960 health care expenditures in the United States rose at approximately the same rate as they did in the other countries of the OECD (Organization for Economic Cooperation and Development), although in recent years the differential has increased somewhat. Interestingly, though, while all of the OECD countries devote smaller percentages of their GNP to health care than does the U.S., some six other countries have had even higher rates of increase of health care expenditures than the U.S. over the last several decades (Figure 2). Some very potent worldwide forces are at work. The key force is technological advance and the particular forms it has taken, forms which were dictated largely by the U.S. incentive structure.

Fact three. The post-World War II era has seen an enormous expansion of health care insurance coverage. Few people in the U.S. had any kind of health care insurance at the onset of the war, and, while coverage expanded during the war, only 9 percent of the population had surgical insurance coverage by 1945. Twenty-five years later 78 percent of citizens had such coverage, and by 1989 the figure was 87 percent (Figure 3).

Year	Hospital Expense Coverage	Surgical Expense Coverage	Health Care Coverage
1940	9	4	
1945	23	9	
1950	50	36	
1955	61	52	
1960	68	62	
1965	71	67	
1970	77	74	
1975	82	78	
1980	83	78	
1985			85
1986			85
1987			86
1988			86
1989			87

Figure 3. Percent of Population Covered by Health Care Insurance 1940–1989 (Selected Years).

Sources: *Source Book of Health Insurance Data 1991*, Table 1.1, page 7; *Source Book of Health Insurance Data 1984–1985*, Table 1.1, page 10; *Economic Report of the President, February 1991*, Table B-31, page 321.

Fact four. The post-World War II era has seen historically un-precedented technological advances. In the case of prescription drugs, for example, as much as 30 percent of the 200 largest-selling drugs are new each year (Figure 4); fully 75 percent of the 200 top-selling drugs in 1972 were gone from the group fifteen years later. Advances in organ transplantation techniques also illustrate the enormity of technological change. During one decade—the 1980s —the number of heart transplants increased from virtually zero to nearly 1,700 per year; liver transplants soared from essentially zero to 2,160 per year.

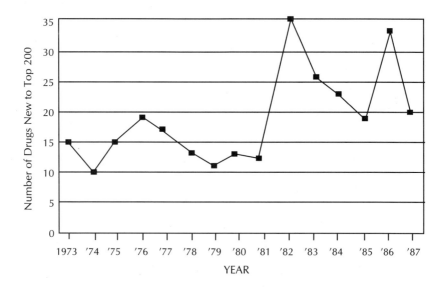

Figure 4. Drugs New to Top 200 from 1973–1987
Based on Number of Prescriptions.
Source: "Drugs New to Top 200," *Pharmacy Times,* 1973 to 1987.

These facts are all interrelated; the extent of insurance coverage, the forms that R&D take, and the level of health care expenditures all reflect the dynamic interplay of incentives. Increased insurance coverage and expanded technology have interacted to drive total health care expenditures upward (Figure 5). The expansion of health care insurance sent a powerful signal to the R&D sector (Fig-ure 6): develop anything that is effective (as urged by physicians, hospitals, or the FDA) and do not be concerned about its cost, be-cause an insurer—private or governmental—will pay. The R&D

sector responded to both incentives. It turned its considerable energy and creativity to the search for ever more effective means to detect and treat, and sometimes to prevent, illness. The R&D sector was enormously successful; but it also disregarded costs. The result was historically unprecedented improvements in health care but also historically unprecedented increases in costs.

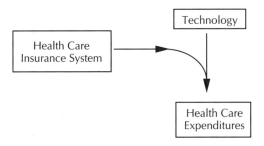

Figure 5. The State of Technology and the Incentives to Use the Technology Determine Total Expenditures: The Short Run.

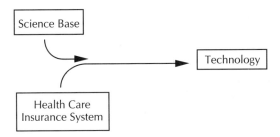

Figure 6. The Health Care Insurance System Establishes Incentives for the R&D Sector.

Just as growing insurance coverage encouraged the development of effective but high-cost technologies, so too was there a reciprocal response. The development of those technologies sent a powerful signal to consumers: obtain even more comprehensive health care insurance or you will be unable to pay for the wonderful but high-cost innovations. Consumers also respond to incentives; they demanded more expansive health insurance coverage from employers and, for the elderly and the poor, from government through Medicare and Medicaid programs (Figure 7).

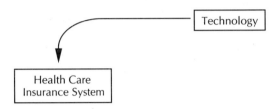

Figure 7. The Technical Capability for Delivering Health Care Affects the Form and Coverage of the Health Care Insurance System.

The system's response was powerful. Expanded health insurance coverage, to more people and to an ever-wider range of technologies, cut consumers' sensitivity to rising costs of care; that expansion signaled for industry to develop costly new technologies, and those new technologies further increased the demand for insurance, which again stimulated R&D aimed at innovations that were medically effective, regardless of cost. And so health care costs soared. As they increased, consumers were under growing pressure to seek expanded insurance coverage (Figure 8).

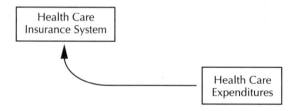

Figure 8. The Level of Health Care Expenditures Affects the Demand for Insurance.

These diagrams may help to portray the health care system that is generating the bulk of health care cost growth. The system is complex, but its components are not. Figure 5 portrays the fact that the level of health care expenditures at any point in time depends largely on the incentives that the insurance system presents to utilize or not utilize the existing technology. Figure 6 shows that the insurance system affects incentives to use the science base to develop new technologies. Figure 7 indicates that the type of health care technology that is available affects the demand for health insurance. Figure 8 shows that changes in health care expenditures cause changes in the demand for insurance. Figure 9 puts these relatively simple subsystems together; simplified as it may be, it portrays the web of key interdependencies among the health insurance system, the R&D system, and the level of health expenditures. Public policy should be constructed in recognition of system-wide ramifications; a change in one element will change the others.

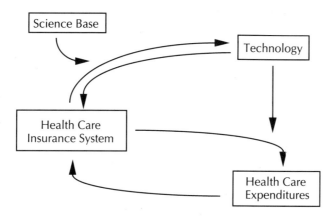

Figure 9. The Dynamic System of Interaction of the Health Care Insurance System, Technological Change, and Health Care Expenditures.

As the United States struggles today with health care policy, there are two important lessons to be learned from the past forty years:

1. The kinds of new technologies developed in recent decades would have taken very different forms if the incentives facing the R&D sector had been different—if, for example, there had been large rewards for developing cost-reducing technologies. Public policy can redirect R&D and thereby stem the upward trajectory of health care costs. The effects of such a redirection of R&D would not be visible immediately—the R&D "pipeline" is typically ten years or more long—but we can begin to turn around incentives now.

2. In health care, as elsewhere, there is no "free lunch"; the

harder we try to contain health care costs, the more we will displace R&D on quality-enhancing therapies. Early evidence indicates that incentives are already beginning to shift away from quality and in favor of holding down costs and prices. Cost-conscious HMOs more than tripled their memberships during the 1980s—from nine million persons in 1980 to nearly twenty-nine million in 1987. In the late 1980s a scientifically promising line of research on a cochlear implant for hearing-impaired persons was discontinued because the downward price pressure emanating from the Medicare Diagnosis Related Group (DRG) hospital-service pricing system was expected to reduce its profitability. Earlier, in the 1970s, when a ceiling price was placed on government payment for kidney dialysis, the direction of R&D was promptly affected in favor of cost reduction: large surface dialyzers were developed that cut the time required per session from the 6 to 8 hour range down to the 3.5 to 4.5 hour range. The point is not that any of these responses to price pressure is undesirable, only that they reflect shifts away from the search for quality in favor of the search for lower cost.

There should be more incentives for health system R&D to develop cost-reducing knowledge. If that is done, we can do more than contain aggregate costs; we can deal with a problem that is seriously dividing our society—the widening gap between the most advanced technologies for health care and the level of care that society is willing to assure to all citizens. Public policy is now in search of a "basic package" of health care services to be guaranteed to our entire population. Few Americans, however, would find it acceptable to define such a package as comprising even the most advanced state of technology in, say, 1960. What is "basic" today depends very much on what is possible today, not on what was possible in the past. The more we develop expensive but effective new technologies, the more the cost of a politically and socially acceptable basic package of services will escalate. The recent experience of the Oregon initiative showed the gargantuan difficulty of reaching consensus on the content of a basic package of health services. Devising a mechanism for expanding the basic package in light of technological change is a challenge that lies just ahead.

It is worthwhile to encourage states to experiment with alternative formulations of the basic services to be made available to everyone. Our longer-term social policy goal, however, should be to focus not on defining a *minimal* level of services but on narrowing the technological *difference* between truly high quality care and the quality that we are willing to make available to all our citizens. Narrowing that gap requires focusing on R&D, and specifically on shifting incentives in favor of developing new technologies that cut costs.

My emphasis on R&D that would be cost reducing should not be confused with the current rush to "technology assessment," which represents the use of cost-effectiveness analysis to determine the desirability of adopting technologies that already have been developed. At that point it is largely too late to focus on costs. Society is tortured by the prospect of facing squarely the question of whether a potentially life-saving technology that already exists is "worth" the cost; *should* society, for example, pay the $300,000 annual cost to treat each victim of certain painful and life-threatening complications of a particular disease treated with a new drug? Should society adopt measures to discourage development of such a costly technology? Or should we encourage R&D on even such high-cost products, but then subsidize their prices to consumers? Or should we force the developers to reduce prices?

How can public policy go about redirecting health care R&D toward cost-reducing technologies? I will indicate a direction we can take; once we accept the central importance of reorienting R&D we can move to the challenge of devising operational programs and incentives.

If we want to send a clear signal to the R&D sector that cutting costs of health care is more important than further improvements in quality—and there is little doubt that this is the trade-off—one idea is to establish large prizes for cost-reducing technologies. Just a few months ago, a consortium of electricity producers offered a $30 million prize for the development of a refrigerator that would reduce electricity usage by 25 percent; two finalists were selected to submit prototypes. With aggregate health care expenditures of $900 billion per year, we can easily consider prizes of hundreds of millions of dollars. This would dramatically increase incentives for the R&D sector. Health care costs would not drop immediately, of course, but society would have taken a vital step toward a meaningful long-term strategy for cost containment.

Making incentives clear is no easy task. A decade ago Medicare instituted the DRG pricing system to help control hospital costs. Hospitals now receive essentially fixed prices for treating a Medicare patient; the payment depends on the person's particular diagnosis, not on the actual costs incurred. The intended incentive was for hospitals to pay more attention to cost control. What kind of incentive does the DRG system send to the R&D sector? The answer is not clear, the reason being that there has been scarcely any policy debate over how the DRG system should respond to the development of new technologies generated by the R&D process. How rigid or how responsive to new technologies will the set of DRGs and their prices be? Depending on the answer, the system will send entirely different incentive signals to the R&D sector. Consider two very different cases. In one, the number of DRG categories and the prices paid by Medicare for each would be fixed permanently. In this case, any device, drug, or technique that was effective but more costly would have a quite limited market, for hospitals would find it difficult to pay for a product that had a greater overall cost of treatment, even if it brought longer life or higher quality of life for the patient. Hospitals would shun cost-increasing innovations.

But what if the DRG regulatory system was very flexible, so that any new medical technology product that was effective would lead to the establishment of a new DRG with a price that was high enough to permit a hospital to adopt it? In this case, the DRG system would devolve into essentially the kind of cost-based reimbursement system that we have had for most of the post-World War II era, and the DRG system would lose its cost-cutting incentive effect.

The United States seems to be traveling a kind of middle road between these extremes, with some new DRG categories having been established and prices to hospitals having been altered. The resulting signal to the R&D sector is less than clear; incentives for R&D on quality-enhancing versus cost-reducing technology are ambiguous.

In summary, society does not have to simply respond to tomorrow's technology; we can shape it. However, as we do so, and, more broadly, as we develop health care policy in its many dimensions, we should bear in mind that the United States is in a unique position among nations. We are both the world's preeminent *producer* of health care R&D and the preeminent *consumer* of its products. For most other nations, changes in their health care insurance systems or in their price policies for health care resources have little or no effect on their own R&D sector, because most have little or no R&D. Similarly, their policies have relatively little effect on the R&D sector of the United States, because each country—although not the aggregate of all countries—constitutes a relatively small market compared with that of the United States. For the U.S., however, health care R&D is both a large and highly successful innovative industry and one that is affected in a major way by our own decisions to encourage or discourage it.

I urge U.S. policymakers to refocus their thinking about health care. R&D is, in my judgment, the driving force behind both the wonderful advances in health care since World War II and the increasingly contentious advances in its costs. But the R&D sector was responding to social incentives operating largely through the health care insurance system. It will respond to new incentives, if we set them clearly and predictably, to give greater emphasis to cost containment. We need a better balance between improving quality and controlling costs. What is the future for health care technology? The answer, in significant measure, remains ours to choose.

Discussion

One discussant noted the increase in numbers of physicians relative to the population, resulting in increased incentives to treat: "If you have a headache, you can either give the patient two aspirins or give them a CAT scan or MRI and two aspirins. Everyone with a headache does not need a CAT scan. I think there is a correlation between the increased number of physicians and the increase in the costs of medical care."

Dr. Weisbrod responded: "Physicians also respond to incentives. There were times when the number of physicians was decreasing relative to the population. We then proceeded to increase the incentive for medical schools to turn out more physicians and, lo and behold, they did. Physicians know that if they see more patients and do more things, they make more money. If we had a system such that physicians would not make more money by seeing more patients, sort of a capitation or HMO approach, the incentives would be completely different. It is important to note that situations facing physicians have changed a great deal in the last generation. Life used to be simpler. The Hippocratic oath basically says, 'Physician, look out for the well-being of your patient.' The physician was the agent for the patient. What has happened in recent decades is that, increasingly, physicians have been put into the position of being agents for the fiscal authority, the gatekeepers. The physician is now in the unenviable position of being a double agent, an incompatible and unenviable situation."

CHAPTER 11

Engineering Cost-Effective Health Care Technologies

DOV JARON
National Science Foundation

"Mobilize the engineering and scientific community to be proactive on the issue, to stimulate the community to ask some serious questions about the role of technology, to provoke new thinking, to raise the awareness of our community, and to hopefully reverse the perception that technology itself or its developers are responsible for the rising costs of health care."

The National Science Foundation (NSF) and the Whitaker Foundation recently announced a new research thrust in cost-effective health care technologies. There were many people involved in making this new thrust possible, particularly NSF's Assistant Director for Engineering, Joe Bordogna, a great believer that technology can be used to help contain health care costs.

Thirty-six million Americans do not have access to health care. There is no question that rising health care costs are affecting each one of us. Every time we visit a physician or are admitted to the hospital the bill becomes more expensive. The increasing costs are affecting both small and large businesses. Some small businesses are closing because they cannot afford to provide health insurance to their employees. The problem is affecting our national economy, our ability to compete in the national market, and (unless something is done about it) it will affect the standard of living of the present generation as well as that of generations to come.

There are several culprits responsible for the rising costs of health care: the third-party payment system, the lack of incentives, exorbitant fees charged by health care providers, excessive litigation (forcing physicians to practice defensive medicine and perform more procedures than are necessary), inefficiencies, and perhaps fraud and waste in the system. There is also a perception, sometimes justified, that medical technology is one of the major drivers of accelerating health care costs; by implication, the creators of those technologies are also to blame. If indeed we have a hand in the rising costs of health care, we should also be part of the solution to rising costs.

Historically technology has always been a major factor in increasing economic efficiency and productivity, in creating national wealth, and in improving the standard of living. But this is not true in the health care system. Technology has not really done much to address the cost issues related to health care. Our profession recently has been talking about the issues involved and discussing ways in which we can become active participants in developing ways in which technology can indeed help to reduce or at least contain health care costs. As a result of those discussions, the National Science Foundation (NSF) and the Whitaker Foundation jointly sponsored a workshop on "Technology for Health Care Cost Containment" in April 1992. The workshop included engineers, physicians, other health care professionals, economists, health care administrators, and representatives from NSF and NIH. The workshop report has been published.[1] The purposes of the workshop were to define areas where engineering and technology can be applied to contain costs and to make general recommendations to NSF and the Whitaker Foundation on the role the two entities can play in this process.

The workshop was followed by a task force formed by NSF, which included representatives from the directorates for engineering, computer information science, and engineering (social, behavioral, and economic), as well as the mathematics and physical sciences directorate. It also included representatives from the Whitaker Foundation and NIH. The outcome was a recommendation for a research thrust jointly funded by NSF and the Whitaker

Foundation called "Cost-Effective Health Care Technologies." We expect that the results of this research will help to contain or reduce costs without compromising the quality of medical care.

The thrust is also intended to function as a catalyst to mobilize the engineering and scientific communities to be proactive on the issue, to stimulate the community to ask some serious questions about the role of technology, to provoke new thinking, to raise the awareness of our community, and, hopefully, to reverse the perception that technology itself or its developers are responsible for the rising costs of health care. It is also intended to stem some of the rhetoric that advocates some curtailment of the development of new medical technologies.

We are certainly not seeking to fund another expensive MRI system or another costly machine to sustain life. That is not our objective. We hope instead to stimulate research to develop new technologies that, in the long run, will enable systemic changes to be made in health care delivery. Clearly, the problem is enormous and we have very modest funds to start this initiative. At this time we can address only a subset of the problem.

We encouraged proposals in three different areas:

1. Technologies that would bring about major changes in the hospital system by increasing efficiency and effectiveness. Examples include the creation of a system that supplies real time, fully integrated monitoring at the bedside; the use of operation research technologies and information and communication technologies; and the development of knowledge-base and other relevant technologies that will change the present paradigm by which care is provided in the hospital setting.

2. Development of technologies that will accelerate the decentralization of the health care delivery system and move it away from the most expensive environment to other areas, such as the home setting. We expect that such changes will reduce the costs without compromising quality. Although this trend has already begun, maintaining the same quality of care requires that new technologies be developed, examples of which include communications and effective networking.

3. Development of technologies which will empower the patient, facilitating reliable self-diagnosis and increasing the ability for self-therapy.

Another emphasis of this thrust is the creation of teams. We would like to bring engineers and scientists together with health care providers in order that the problems they address are problems on which both sides agree. NSF does not fund any clinical work, so the research proposals that come to us cannot directly involve patients.

The NSF-Whitaker research thrust on cost-effective health care technology was announced in March 1993; it resulted in more than 100 formal proposals. For further information, contact:

Bioengineering Program
Biological and Critical Systems Division
The National Science Foundation
1800 G Street, NW
Washington, DC 20550
Phone: 202–357–9545
FAX: 202–357–9803

The Whitaker Foundation
901 15th St. NW
Suite 100
Washington, DC 20005
Phone: 202–833–6920
Fax: 202–833–6928
Email: P00019@PSILINK.COM

References

1. J.D. Andrade, D. Jaron, and P. Katona, "Improved Delivery and Reduced Costs of Health Care Through Engineering," *IEEE Engineering in Medicine and Biology Magazine* (June, 1993): 38–41.

CHAPTER 12

Initiatives in Biomedical Technologies

RICHARD SATAVA
Advanced Research Projects Agency (ARPA)

"ARPA has a vision of how medicine may be changed in the future."

"Telepresence refers to manipulating remote objects in the real world, whereas virtual reality creates its own world in which you can merge yourself and manipulate the objects within it.... Telepresence surgery...will help the surgeon by giving 3-D vision, dexterity, and sensation back to his or her hands."

"Your resident can practice safely on a computer without fear of AIDS or other contamination, without the fear of animal-rights concern."

"Multiple surgeons could operate upon one patient at the same time through two telepresence systems."

"Bring the surgeon right to the battlefield, right at the time of wounding, but using telepresence."

ARPA has a vision of how medicine may be changed in the future. Why did ARPA and the Department of Defense (DOD) get into the biomedical technology arena? Defense has two responsibilities. The first is to the individual soldier by minimizing and treating battle casualties. Throughout this century, despite improvements in technology, we have not been able to decrease battle casualties on the front line; we still sustain 90 percent of our casualties in the front lines. As the DOD redefines its role away from traditional military confrontations, it now has taken on humanitarian responsibilities. Individual soldiers are now assuming strategic as well as tactical importance. For example, in Somalia, that single marine who was wounded during the humanitarian effort had an international impact, one well beyond his importance as a tactical soldier. The second responsibility of the DOD is to peacetime health care; one of the largest HMOs in the United States is the Military Medical System of the Department of Defense.

At its creation in 1958 ARPA was envisioned as *the* national technology engine, with the responsibility of finding new and innovative technologies and maintaining and enhancing the nation's technological edge in medicine and health care. We propose to exploit this technological edge. There is no question that we can deploy these technological advantages for dual use, whether they be for innovative treatment modalities, diagnostics, and medical informatics, or for advanced education and training environments. We will not be looking into the areas of policy and cost savings per se, but developments in those areas will be a result of the work we do.

Several thrusts have already matured within ARPA. One is the global grid—a global telecommunications infrastructure which will permit integrated medical-informatics programs. We expect to provide a support structure for medical devices, the development of personal status monitors, telesurgery, and medicine—all built upon the information infrastructure in the global grid.

There are many nonmedical technologies that have come from business, industry, and academia. The vast majority of things that have been medical improvements have not originated from "medical" research; they have been technologies that we have inherited and adapted to the medical field. In addition, we have now a new technology, laparoscopic surgery, a minimally invasive surgical procedure. Until recently all operations were performed by literally ripping the patient open, manipulating his/her organs, removing those that were damaged, repairing them, and then putting the patient back together again. Today that process is not necessary for many procedures, because we can make tiny holes, insert small cameras and instruments, and remove or repair the organs without ever having to cut the patient open. This has been an absolutely giant step forward for the patient, who has decreased pain, is often out of the hospital in a day, and is back to work in a week, instead of being in the hospital for a week and back to work in six weeks. Yet, while this has been a giant leap forward for the patient, it has been three giant steps backward for the surgeons. We have lost our 3-D vision, our sense of touch, and we no longer have the dexterity that we had during the open procedure.

We have a new type of surgeon coming on the scene—our children. The ones that you and I are concerned about because they have been playing too much Nintendo. Well, they are the new surgeons of the future and they have a new skill, something that you and I did not have intuitively as we grew up. They are able to look at a television screen or monitor and are able to manipulate things on it. At this time it may be only PacMan eating bugs, but in the future it may be the ability to perform surgery remotely. The pivotal event and driving force for this change was laparoscopic surgery. It has had a profound effect upon the way medicine is being performed today. Yet, despite its benefit to the patient, surgeons want their 3-D vision, sense of touch, and dexterity back. We have explored several areas and have been able to put together a framework for the future of surgery, applicable to medicine as a whole.

Virtual reality may indeed be at the heart of one of the most profound changes that we have been able to discover. Consider a surgical workstation not too dissimilar from today's radiology workstation. By using telepresence, networking, robotic control, and artificial intelligence, we will be able to enhance the power of the surgeon. The world of virtual realty not only will bring training and education but also will bring in planning as well as prognostication. Virtual reality as we know it today requires a helmet with stereoscopic TV cameras in front and earphones that isolate you from the real world. Once you put on the helmet, the only thing you are aware of is what the computer presents. A virtual world is not a real world, but one has the sensation that it is real. Imagine a glove (called the "gesture input device") replacing a joystick. This would allow you to roam around inside the imaginary world, grab things, pick them up, and move them as if they actually existed.

With virtual reality we can practice on things that don't really exist but have the potential for existing. A person in a virtual world is completely isolated from everything, working within this imaginary world almost like Alice in Wonderland down in the rabbit hole. In about 1940 Edwin Link came forward with the first airplane simulator, and we all know how important flight simulators are today. Pilots never even get into aircraft until they spend hundreds or thousands of hours with flight simulators and have perfected their techniques. Virtual reality is on that cusp. Consider a virtual reality surgical simulator. But there is a difference between telerobotics, telepresence, and virtual reality. Virtual reality is an imaginary world, whereas telepresence is in the real world.

Teleoperation involves a remote hand controlled by the operator on a one-to-one basis. As the operator moves his or her hand, the remote slave hand moves. This is very distinct from telerobotics. In telerobotics there is also a remote manipulating hand, but that hand is controlled by robotics—it has an independent knowledge of its own. Telepresence is akin to teleoperation in the sense that it is a one-to-one relationship between one's hand and the remote arm. The new technology of virtual reality has some similarities to telepresence. Telepresence refers to manipulating remote objects in the real world, whereas virtual reality creates its own world in which one can merge and manipulate the objects within it. What does this have to with surgery? There are at least two things: education and basic surgical anatomy, as well as training a surgeon to operate.

In learning anatomy one could use a virtual reality surgical simulator to actually travel inside of the organs and learn new perspectives about how the human anatomy should be perceived, perspectives one couldn't possibly get even if you dissect a cadaver. You could fly through the stomach into the duodenum, back up the bile duct and out the gallbladder. One of the interesting things about the virtual world is that you can enlarge or become microscopic in size depending upon the perspective you want. Currently all we are able to do is operate on individual organs that are large enough for us to see. But there are a number of disease states in which we may want to go down to small organs or even to the cellular level.

Pilots for past generations have been learning how to fly by using flight simulators. They have not been allowed to fly an aircraft until they have performed and perfected their aviation techniques on a simulator. A virtual reality simulator will provide the interactions, feelings, and 3-D aspects of being in an operative procedure, but without one ever having to touch a patient. Your resident can practice safely on a computer without fear of AIDS or other contamination, and without the fear of animal-rights concerns. A simulator has all of these educational and training potentials. In addition, it can be a powerful research tool. Today, architects can show their building drawings in 3-D and can go through them with their clients. There is no reason why we cannot, with a properly created anatomy, do surgical research without ever having to operate on an animal. These are potentials and benefits that were well beyond anyone's imagination as few as five to ten years ago. There is no reason why virtual reality simulation shouldn't be pursued aggressively; it is done in all other areas of industry and technology. Medicine should catch up. This technology will be absolutely integral to new foundations of surgery and medicine; education, training, surgery, and post-procedure evaluation will all be part of a single, seamless system.

We should be doing telepresence surgery.[1] Telepresence surgery was developed as an answer to laparoscopic surgery. It will help the surgeon by giving 3-D vision, dexterity, and sensation back to his or her hands. For example, after the surgeon initially puts in the trochar, s/he will sit next to the patient. This is a natural transition from laparoscopic surgery and has the advantage of giving the surgeon the feeling of being in an open operative procedure. As it is performed, what we have is a connection between the patient and surgeon via an "umbilical cord." With laparoscopic surgery, we are removing internal organs without ever actually seeing them or touching them. What we do is look at the TV screen, take an instrument and stab it in the belly, and hope that what we are poking at is actually what we are seeing on the screen. By doing this with telepresence, we will in essence be able to put an electronic interface between the surgeon and patient that will enhance the surgeon's abilities. By having that interface, we also will be able to bring other things to bear as well. For example, if we operate from a surgical workstation, we don't have to be in the same place as the patient. Two or more surgeons could operate upon one patient at the same time through two telepresence systems.

We could have a medical center—in essence, the medical center of the future, the medical center without walls—using telemedicine, whether it be teleradiology, telesurgery, or video consultation. Such a medical center could reach out to remote, small clinics, embracing those remote clinics as part of their actual system, and multiply the power and effect of each individual physician, particularly the specialist. Small communities would have access to the care that is now only available within our urban medical centers. We could provide services to places that are too remote or dangerous to get to—such as space stations or third world countries, for example. Assuming that we have the surgical workstation, or physician's workstation, we will not only be able to incorporate real time and real patient care but also we will be able to bring 3-D images, MRI, and CT scans, and superimpose them upon the actual patient being operated upon, thus giving the surgeon real time, x-ray "vision" while s/he is operating. S/he will be able to see, deeply imbedded in the liver, that cancerous lesion because of the 3-D projection of the CT scan or the MRI.

A surgical simulator brings realistic images to the surgeon in training identical to what s/he would see on real people.[2] S/he practices on the computer simulation and with the flip of a switch can perform surgery on a real patient. We will then have flattened out the learning curve. The surgeon does not have to practice on a plastic model or an animal in training, and then be supervised. S/he will be able to do this in a single step. Finally, this technology is not limited to surgical procedures. Other procedures, such as endoscopy and microsurgery, will be possible from remote workstations.

The DOD believes strongly that this concept is worthy of being pushed forward by the soldier of the future (Figure 1). The conceptual interaction between the soldier of the future and medicine of the future developed because we realized that we will have to monitor the soldier at all times. Imagine soldiers on the battlefield with personal status monitors on their wrists or collars providing continuous real time vital signs, their location on the battlefield, and whether or not they are friendly forces. When a soldier is wounded, this individual will set up an alert on the global system over the global grid so that anyone will be able to know that s/he is wounded and precisely where s/he is located. Medics rapidly can go to the casualty and remote telepresence surgery can be performed via a mobile armored van (Figure 1).

In ancient times, battle casualties were taken care of after the battle. When the battle was over, the surgeon would go out and fix what he could while everybody else was back home eating. In 1796

Dominique Larrey revolutionized battle casualty care in medicine with the ambulance. Now when the soldier was wounded he was immediately evacuated to a field hospital. There was still a time delay, however, called the "golden hour of surgery." Our intent is to bring the surgeon right to the battlefield, right at the time of wounding, but using telepresence. In addition, the information that is going to be available from the personal status monitor to the medics will be distributed so that all necessary individuals will have that information available to them.

The ARPA perspective is that the grand challenge to revolutionize the delivery of health care lies with the electronic interface. This will be enabled by

- the Health Care Information Infrastructure; and
- High Performance Computing and Communications (HPCC), of which the global grid telecommunications network is critical.

With these two ARPA programs well on the way to maturity, the Biomedical Technology Program will fund projects in the following areas:

1. Advanced diagnostics, including remote sensing of vital signs (such as the Personal Status Monitor), portable miniature "stat labs," advanced digital imaging devices of all types (CT, MRI, PET, SPECT, ultrasound, surface laser scanning), telemedicine consultations (such as teleradiology, telepathology, etc.).

2. Advanced interventional therapy, including telepresence surgery, pharmacologic agents (against shock/hemorrhage which can be autoinjected at the time of injury), and Trauma Pod to provide complete stabilization and en route therapy during evacuation.

3. Advanced training and evaluation, limited to using advanced simulation technologies, such as virtual environments to permit virtual prototyping of equipment, virtual training on a simulated "cadaver," or medical forces training in the SIMNET environment.

4. Medical information infrastructure, which will include massive medical data bases, shared/distributed environments which are platform independent, and decision support (such as a "Medic or Physician Associate").

What is common to all of the above projects is that they are *all* mediated through a digital interface (even the pharmacologic

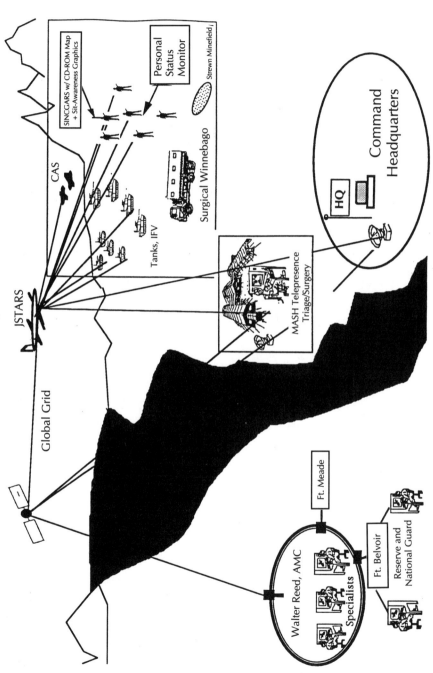

Figure 1: The Modern Medical Battlefield.

agents are to be administered using some form of digitally controlled device). The revolution is the digital physician and the advanced technologies which will enhance the physician's abilities. There will be advanced technology demonstrations in 1995 and 1997 to showcase these new technologies in a military environment which is linked to the civilian sector (dual use). Wisely implementing the above technologies will give us leverage to actually decrease the costs of health care.

References

1. P.S. Green, J.H. Hill, and R.M. Satava, "Telepresence: Dextrous Procedures in a Virtual Operating Field," (abstract) *Surgical Endoscopy* 57(1991): 192.

P.S. Green, R.M. Satava, and I.B. Simon, "Telepresence: Advanced Teleoperator Technology for Minimally Invasive Surgery," (abstract) *Surgical Endoscopy* 6(1992): 90.

R.M. Satava and P.S. Green, "The Next Generation: Telepresence Surgery. Current Status and Implications for Endoscopy," (abstract) *Gastro-intestinal Endoscopy* 38(1992): 277.

P.S. Green, R.M. Satava, and I.B. Simon, "Telepresence: Advanced Teleoperator Technology for Minimally Invasive Surgery," (abstract) *Surgical Endoscopy* 6(1992): 90.

R.M. Satava, "Robotics, Telepresence and Virtual Reality: A Critical Analysis of the Future of Surgery," *Minimally Invasive Therapy* 1(1992): 357–63.

R.M. Satava, "Speculation on Future Technology" in J.G. Hunter and J.E. Sakier. *High Tech Surgery: New Approaches to Old Diseases* (New York: McGraw Hill, 1993), 339–47.

2. R.M. Satava, "Surgery 2001: A Technologic Framework for the Future," *Surgical Endoscopy* 7(1993): 111–13.

R.M. Satava, "Virtual Reality Surgical Simulator: The First Steps," *Surgical Endoscopy* 7(1993): 203–5.

CHAPTER 13

National Initiatives for the Enhancement of Information and Communication

MICHAEL NELSON
Office of Science and Technology Policy

"A sense of geological time scales...is very useful in dealing with Congress."

"We are moving ahead aggressively.... We will have the core technology from which to build the rest of the infrastructure."

"Help schools and other information have-nots get into the information game."

"We have to find new ways to fund the research and development that develops the new technologies that underly the new products and the new jobs."

"It is a very exciting time to be involved in the political process. Geological political time has sped up."

"Scientists have had a method of picking subjects and problems for over five hundred years which has been exceedingly successful. If we replace that with political methods, such as priority setting, we are unlikely to do better, and will most certainly do worse." (C. McDonald)

I have been impersonating Senator Gore for several years, and now I get to impersonate Vice President Gore. I guess that is a promotion. I am a geologist by training; after finishing a Ph.D. at MIT, I came down to the Hill on a one-year fellowship, thinking that it would be an interesting detour before going back to a career in research. I quickly learned to enjoy working on science policy and stayed on. One reason was that, as a geologist, I was very well trained for work in science policy—I had a sense of geological time scales, which is very useful in dealing with Congress. I have been working on information technology issues for several years, and it has been one of the more exciting things I have done.

I am now in the White House Office of Science and Technology Policy (OSTP). Before that, I worked in the vice president's office trying to help the new administration put together its budget for science and technology. In the next few years I will be working with Dr. John Gibbons, the director of OSTP, with Vice President Gore, and with people in the agencies to implement our vision of an information infrastructure.

This chapter briefly outlines our information technology programs and suggests how they can benefit the biomedical engineering community. It also asks how the community can assist in developing this initiative to make sure it meets the needs of the community and the health care needs of all Americans.

When we were developing Senator Gore's legislation on high-performance computing in 1990–91, the medical applications of the advanced computing technology were always of great interest. Senator Gore's legislation set up the high-performance computing and communications program (HPCC), which provided funding to develop more advanced supercomputers and more advanced software to run on those supercomputers, high-speed networks to allow people to interact across the distances, and training for the people who will develop and use the next generation of information technology. It was a very broad bill. In one of the first hearings we held on high-performance computing there were graphic demonstrations of CAT scans of the brain, processed to develop a 3-D model which could be manipulated in electronic space. The fact that we can look at things in 3-D and then process the data any way we please makes the program a very powerful tool. The idea that we can use information technology in this way helped bring home the message that the billions of dollars we are proposing to spend in this area are going to provide multiple benefits in health care and other fields.

Another very exciting application is the ability to use high-speed networks to provide medical services to rural communities and to other areas well away from major medical centers. The idea that a family doctor in a small town in South Dakota would be able to use a high-speed network to teleconfer with a specialist at the Mayo Clinic and share CAT scan imagery and other data with that doctor to get a second opinion had a lot of appeal to the members of our committee—partly because about 60 percent of them were from rural states like South Dakota.

Medical records is another exciting area (see Horn, Chapter 7; and McDonald, Chapter 15). If we can have more powerful supercomputers, better databases, high-speed networks, and then be able to connect them all, we can really save money on medical records. In consolidating those records by putting them all in electronic form, you eliminate the need for acres of filing cabinets and the need for transferring records between different doctors' offices. You also eliminate problems with lost or misplaced records. According to some estimates, use of technologies like these could actually cut the total federal bill for health care by between 20 and 60 billion dollars a year. That is pretty substantial, and the idea raised a lot of eyebrows among the senators.

Another area where high-performance computing would be useful is in the sequencing of DNA. One of the biggest challenges for the Human Genome Initiative is how to quickly and effectively store and process all the genetic information that will come out of that project. How do you match the sequences; how do you find what you really need?

Another area is epidemiology. If we can do a better job of collecting medical records and outcomes, we can do a better job of determining where the pressing health concerns are. Are there regional differences that we need to understand and address? There are many different areas where more advanced computing and more advanced networking can help, and health care is certainly one area where we can save the country hundreds of billions of dollars.

President Clinton has released a technology plan as part of his economic plan. He and Vice President Gore visited Silicon Graphics, a computer firm in Silicon Valley, where they released a 36-page policy paper to provide a framework for technology. It was released online at the same time the president was releasing it in California. The area of information infrastructure is one of six new initiatives in the plan and is a concept that appears throughout the policy document. The document has two parts. One is a framework which brings order to the entire federal technology effort; the other consists of the six initiatives, one of which is information infrastructure.

The first objective is to adequately fund and implement the high-performance computing and communications program. This program has been in place for several years and has focused on developing the core technologies: faster supercomputers, more sophisticated software, faster networks. Most of the work is being done at ARPA, the Advanced Research Projects Agency; NSF, which primarily funds university research; the Department of Energy, which is using its federal labs to develop technology; and NASA, which has a key role to play in high-performance computing and in developing software for aerospace applications. Other important agencies related to the project include the NLM at NIH, the National Institute of Standards and Technology, NOAA at the Department of Commerce, the EPA, and the Department of Education. These participants will help ensure that the new technology can be used by a broad community.

That program is going ahead. We have requested an additional 47 million dollars in fiscal year 1993 to provide additional funding to the NSF so it can fully implement its part of the program. About 850 million dollars is going into this program in 1993 and about a billion dollars in 1994. So we are moving ahead aggressively. Clearly we will have the core technology from which to build the rest of the infrastructure.

The second initiative is the information infrastructure technology program. This is a program focused on taking the technology developed by HPCC and making it user-friendly, accessible to the average American. We will focus on developing applications for advanced computing and networking in four areas: the first is education, not just K through 12 but lifelong learning, including retraining in the workplace; the second area is manufacturing—high-speed networks and supercomputers can do a great deal to help American companies be more competitive in the marketplace and quicker at marketing new products and thus beating their competitors overseas.

The third area is health care. NIH will be the lead agency in developing a range of applications using the core technology. Applications will be developed for rural medicine and telemedicine. NIH will develop technology for handling genetic data, medical records, imagery, and the visualization of medical imagery, such as CAT scans, PET scans, and x rays (see Chapter 14).

The fourth area is libraries, an area that hasn't received enough attention. Vice President Gore is very fond of saying that one of the reasons he is doing all this is so that his son can come home from school and sit down at a device, hopefully no more complicated and no more expensive than a Nintendo machine, and log onto an electronic version of the Library of Congress. This would allow him to see images, hear sounds, and watch videos containing different types of information. He can explore dinosaurs one day, airplanes the next, and cruise through information like you would in a library, picking up a book here and there, examining and exploring and learning new things. It would be a powerful new tool for a child to use to educate himself or herself in many ways, and to get excited about fields of study. The library program would help develop the technology needed to store trillions of bits of data and to make that data accessible to people around the country. We have requested 47 million dollars for 1993 applications to be distributed between NIH, NASA, NSF, and other agencies.

A third part of the overall program is the pilot project program of the Department of Commerce. We want to use the federal government to help schools, libraries, and other nonprofit organizations explore what they can do with networking. There are a lot of schools that would love to get on Internet and connect up to the world, but they don't have the money to get a few computers and a modem. This program is designed to help schools and other information have-nots get into the information game and take advantage of the network and technology that is out there. This program will start off at 47 million dollars and will grow to about 150 million dollars over the next two to three years. It is part of the public telecommunications facilities program at the National

Telecommunications and Information Administration of the Commerce Department. It is a way for the government to demonstrate what is possible, to show people how we can pull it all together and start building these networks. It is really a way to help create an incentive in the private sector to get them in the business of providing these services, and thus drive down the prices and create the momentum needed to build a national high-speed computer network, Gore's long-term goal.

We are moving towards a world in which we will have a high-speed network capable of carrying about a thousand times more information than our present telephone network does and delivering it at about the same cost to every home in America. That is the long-term goal. These programs will help provide the catalyst: by developing the technology, demonstrating that technology, making it accessible to people, and hopefully getting the private sector to step in and move forward. Unfortunately, that will not happen unless we do the fourth part of this initiative, reform our telecommunications policies. We now have a number of regulatory policies that were designed in the 1950s that are just not working. In order to accelerate the technology we have organized an interagency task force to take a close look at where the problems are and then change those regulations which delay the implementation and deployment of this new technology.

The fifth area is information policy. The federal government spends billions of dollars every year collecting information. Unfortunately, it doesn't do a very good job of returning that information to the taxpayers who pay for it. Our hope is that by changing the way we price data, by changing the incentives we give our agencies, we can help get data out to people. NLM has done a very good job of putting medical information on line—other agencies could follow their lead. In so many cases it seems that the pc icy is one of controlling rather than disseminating information.

The fiscal 1994 budget, although greatly constrained, will provide increased funding for these initiatives. In addition to the information infrastructure component of technology policy, there are a number of other exciting pieces. We have devoted significant amounts of additional funding to the Department of Commerce for the commercialization of new technologies. DOC will become a focal point for the development of new technologies. Just as we have had ARPA at the Defense Department for developing technologies for the defense sector, we need the equivalent on the civilian side.

The National Institute of Standards and Technology (NIST) has been chosen as the focal point. The administration is proposing to double the budget for NIST over the next five years. It is going to provide a very dramatic increase for the "Advanced Technology Program," which will provide hundreds of millions of dollars to companies in the form of matching grants for developing new technologies. We are not trying to help someone develop a product but rather to develop a technology and to lay the foundation so that others can go forward and develop something for the marketplace. This really is competitive research. It is the stuff that you can't make money on but which you have to do if you are going to develop new products. It used to be that Bell Labs did that; and the DOD did that, but the money is not there anymore. We have to find new ways to fund the research and development that develops the new technologies that underly the new products and the new jobs.

The Advanced Technology Program has already been funding biomedical technologies, operating much the same way as the NSF—that is, with a broad general announcement of opportunity. We don't want to fund projects that are not going to work or for which there is no market. Our reviews are done primarily by people working in the private sector. NSF and NIH have funded the best basic research in the world because we have a very effective system for funding the best basic research. We want to do the same thing for technology. We are asking companies to put up at least 50 percent of the money—so this becomes a way to help companies that are really willing to work.

Another area of importance is the Clinton administration's broad view of our health care system; we are trying to determine just what it is we can do to drive down the costs of health care. Anybody who has seen the projections knows that we just can't afford the steady growth in health care costs that are projected for the future. One obvious place is telemedicine, with which one specialist can serve a large area. We won't need to have quite so many clinics and hospitals throughout the country, thus saving money.

Medical records is another good example, and one that is getting a great deal of attention. Another area of interest is the national performance review, which President Clinton has announced and which is under Vice President Gore's direction. We are examining the entire federal government from top to bottom, evaluating how it works, how it doesn't work, finding out where the inefficiencies are, finding out how we can do a better job of serving our customers, taxpayers, voters, and children of this country. The performance review also will obviously look at things like the VA hospitals and will touch on some of the same issues that Hillary Clinton's task force looked at. We really have to see how we can better organize our medical agencies and how we can better deliver cost-effective solutions to medical problems.

This is a very exciting time to be involved in the political process. Geological political time has sped up. Things are happening. There are a number of places where biomedical engineering should be involved: for example, in the high-performance computing program, particularly the information infrastructure and technology part. This will develop applications for health care. There hasn't been enough work done on exactly where the benefits are, or on what the potential is of computer technology in health care. There are good people doing good things, but there hasn't been a systematic look at what is going on.

There are a number of groups, inside and outside of government, evaluating the cost-benefit ratios. Where can we do the best job of applying this technology? Where should we put our money? This is primarily the responsibility of the Commerce Department. People who are developing new technologies on the medical side should talk with the Advanced Technology Program at NIST. They are taking a $67-million program and expanding it very rapidly to a nearly $300-million program. It is important that they realize that there are great opportunities in this field and that they should be looking to this sector when making announcements on different programs. OSTP will continue to have a very important role in this development. Dr. John Gibbons, OSTP's director, is very open and eager to find out what is going on out there. He and I will be looking for the advice of the bioengineering community on overall technology policy.

Discussion

There were a number of comments indicating that it may be difficult to develop the money for a national information infrastructure and that existing big technology/big science projects should be reconsidered by the administration, including the strategic defense initiative, the space station, and the superconducting supercollider. Dr. Nelson noted that those projects are being downsized and that funds for all three have been substantially decreased and/or restructured in the last twelve months. There was also a plea to not sacrifice the funding of basic science for such technological initiatives. Nelson projected that it is unlikely that there will be significant increases in basic research but it is also unlikely that there will be significant cuts. He said the administration is happy with the basic-research system, but mentioned that we may need to set priorities better and otherwise improve the process.

Concern was expressed that NSF, and perhaps NIH, is being forced to deal with technology at the expense of their programs in basic science. The questioner expressed concern that the administration may not fully understand the difference between science and technology. Part of Nelson's response dealt with the blurring between science and technology, particularly in biotechnologies and medical sciences. In response to this discussion, Dr. McDonald said that he was disturbed to hear the justification for science being based solely on curiosity. "There is nothing wrong with curiosity," he said, "but I am afraid we have done wrong to say that science should get what it wants because scientists should be allowed to follow their curiosity. Rather, the point is that for over five hundred years scientists have had a method of picking subjects and problems which has been exceedingly successful. If we replace that with political methods, such as priority-setting, we are unlikely to do better, and will almost certainly do worse."

Another questioner noted that there is a big difference between basic molecular biology and the bioprocess engineering that is required to fully apply and commercialize its important developments. Another comment was made to the effect that, although there has been considerable discussion in the administration as to the importance of infrastructure, there appears to have been less emphasis on people infrastructure, i.e., appropriate training and fellowship programs.

PART IV

·

INFORMATION AND COMMUNICATION TECHNOLOGIES

CHAPTER 14

The Information Infrastructure of Health Care

DONALD LINDBERG
Director, National Library of Medicine and Director, National Coordination Office for High Performance Computing and Communication (HPCC)

"The infrastructure of medicine is schools and brains. Traditional medical education has tried to pack the head of a student with all that he or she needs to know in order to practice medicine."

"The importance of lifelong learning is recognized in 1993 legislation that expands the HPCC Program."

"But biology and medicine depend upon more than words. Much of the understanding of complicated processes of health and disease lies in images."

"Digital telecommunications may provide 'agile medical care' via instantaneous video consultation with colleagues at distant major medical centers."

It is clear that the information infrastructure of health care depends on new computer and communications technologies. I believe in computing and communications systems. I took the job with the Office of High Performance Computing and Communication (HPCC) because I believe it to be the most important science project that I have encountered in almost ten years in government.

The infrastructure of medicine is schools and brains. Traditional medical education has tried to pack the head of a student with all that he or she needs to know in order to practice medicine. Although we know that the half-life of medical education is only five years, I am not aware of a single medical school in the United States that teaches lifelong learning—which is the only way physicians can stay current.

We know that computers are the only possible way to provide all the information physicians need. But we don't really equip our physicians to benefit fully from this information technology. Few medical schools in the U.S. even teach students how to use a personal computer.

We all want to be able to deliver information at the time and place that it is needed for patient care. Health care information must be problem-oriented and understandable. The National Library of Medicine (NLM) is the largest source of health care information in the world. Each region of the country has a regional library and many resource libraries, which are networked with 4,000 basic biomedical libraries. Outreach has long been a top priority of the NLM. Outreach means helping health professionals to see how modern information services can make them more effective as health care providers, and it also means lowering the barriers to access that information. Today MEDLINE and the more than forty other databases that make up a system called MEDLARS (Medical Literature Analysis and Retrieval System) comprise the largest and most widely used biomedical computer system in the world. By all measures, the MEDLARS system has been a spectacular success, the only practical way that a biomedical researcher or health care practitioner can keep up with the vast literature in the life sciences. Over 350,000 new articles are entered into the system each year.

NLM's user-friendly computer program—Grateful Med—allows a health professional or researcher to compose a database search in the office or home by simply filling in a form displayed on the computer screen. The program then automatically connects to the NLM computers across high-speed networks, conducts the search, and downloads the results to the user's own computer. Over 50,000 copies of this freely copyable program have been sold, and the majority of searches of NLM databases now are conducted via this user-friendly software.

Grateful Med provides access not only to MEDLINE but also to a growing number of specialized information databank collections on topics such as AIDS, cancer treatment, bioethics, and toxicology. Extensive data on the medical and environmental effects of hazardous chemicals is available via the TOXNET collection of databases, which include recommendations on the management of emergency spills and other environmental releases.

Our "Loansome Doc" program allows for interlibrary loans of articles, which can be delivered by fax or mail, or can be picked up in person at the library. More than five million computer searches were done on the NLM computer system this past year. We know that about half of those searches were done to get information for the direct care of sick patients; the other half were done for medical research and education.

Continuing-education requirements for physicians can range from zero hours in seventeen states to more than thirty-five hours in other locales. For lawyers, more than half of the state bars require continuing education. These requirements range from twelve to fifteen hours. For registered professional engineers, only two states required continuing education—Iowa and Alabama, each of which requires fifteen hours per year. A growing number of engineering specialty groups are beginning to require continuing education; these include the American Academy of Environmental Engineers and the National Academy of Forensic Engineers. Among the fifteen professional societies that comprise AIMBE, none require continuing education for their membership.

The importance of lifelong learning is recognized in the 1993 legislation that expands the HPCC Program. Originally introduced by former Senator Al Gore in 1992, the legislation calls for applications in the areas of health care, education, lifelong learning, digital libraries, and manufacturing. To this end, the HPCC Program recently added a fifth component, Information Infrastructure Applications and Technology (IITA). IITA will support integrated-systems technology for critical applications through development of intelligent systems interfaces, including support for virtual reality, image understanding, and language and speech understanding programs, as well as data and object bases for electronic libraries and commerce.

The original four components of the HPCC Program focused on:

- hardware design,
- the National Research and Education Network (NREN),
- software development, and
- training and education.

Ten federal agencies participate in the program, which had 1993 funding of $800 million.

One of the most visible and successful parts of the HPCC Program is the NREN (National Research and Education Network), the federal core of the Internet. An estimated 1.5 million computers worldwide are connected to the Internet, about 70 percent of which are in the U.S. Approximately 100 countries are connected by the Internet; and more than 1,000 universities and colleges and an additional 1,000 high schools in the U.S. are connected to the Internet.

In terms of the number of addressable networks—not persons, and not computers, but networks—we estimated that by 1993 there would be 10,000. However, before the 1993 year is half over, we are already at 12,500 networks. Some networks encompass entire states, some networks are regional; there is substantial geographical overlap. When the present Internet began in 1987, it connected six supercomputer centers on a backbone that operated at a then phenomenal 1.45 million bits per second. Now the backbone operates at 45 million bits per second. In the future, we will rely upon a backbone transmission speed of greater than a billion bits per second. The number of packets on the network backbone continues to grow by about 12 percent per month. In 1987 the heaviest day occurred when one million packets were on the backbone. The busiest day in 1992 was a billion packets.

But biology and medicine depend upon more than words. Much of the understanding of complicated processes of health and disease lies in images—pictures of body systems, organs, and molecules which cannot effectively be described in words. A standard black-and-white chest x ray may contain the equivalent of at least 32 million points of light, or pixels. We can and do make electronic versions of such medical images at the NLM, but to transmit these images over currently available computer networks is simply not feasible. It would take more than ten hours to send just one x-ray picture. We need an advanced national information infrastructure capable of quickly transmitting these and other forms of computer-based medical information.

For practitioners who work in isolated rural areas, digital tele-communications may provide "agile medical care" via instantaneous video consultation with colleagues at distant major medical centers; or it may also provide the simultaneous viewing of x rays and discussion of findings while both practitioners see the images on viewing screens, perhaps thousands of miles apart.

The National Coordination Office for High Performance Computing and Communications has operated since September 1992 at the National Library of Medicine (phone 301–402–4100; fax 301–402–4080; E-mail nco@hpcc.gov). Its three major functions are to provide: liaison to industry, universities, and Congress; coordination of HPCC Programs across federal agencies; and information about the HPCC Program to all. We would be happy to receive your suggestions.

Discussion

It was noted that second-year medical students seem to have difficulty appreciating the relevance and potential of medical informatics. Dr. Lindberg suggested that fourth-year students might have a very different view—after the students have some clinical experience, they are generally more appreciative of the importance of adequate information sources and infrastructures. There was a brief reference to the Iliad hospital information and medical informatics programs used in many medical schools (Applied Informatics, Inc., Salt Lake City, Utah).

CHAPTER 15

Computer-Stored Medical Records: What They Can Do for Us and What We Should Do for Them

CLEMENT J. MCDONALD, M.D.
Indiana University School of Medicine
Regenstrief Institute for Health Care

"The practice of medicine is still in the hunting-and-gathering stage of social evolution. . . . The computer-based medical record can solve these logistic problems, advancing us to the agricultural stage or beyond."

"Most medicine aims at managing a patient's illness. This is a continuous control effort, and having a stream of data available over time is an important input to refining the care process."

"Sociology is as influential as science in some medical decisions."

"We will be able to see patterns in these data that lead to the discovery of clinical truths and better management of the whole process of care."

Copyrighted material © 1994; *Medical and Biological Engineering in the Future of Health Care*, edited by J.D. Andrade; University of Utah Press.

"You must do a controlled trial to learn anything. This is not universally true.

"It is clear that being alive can get you sued."

"The large regional or national utilization of medical-patient records certainly requires a national information infrastructure."

The computer-based patient record (CPR) will be the most pervasive and influential technology in the future of health care.[1] We often describe the CPR as a computer-stored version of the paper chart; but that understates its capabilities. It would only be accurate if a paper chart could tell you where it was when you called for it, have an intelligent conversation with you regarding the patient's course of treatment, and jump into a pile of paper charts from institutions all over the city to produce useful medical statistics.

Computer medical-record systems will help care by:
- solving the logistic problems of locating and transporting data;
- influencing the care process by providing feedback and intelligent responses to the data they contain; and
- providing new medical insights by enabling us to examine outcomes across the entire population of patients.

These three aspects can be illustrated by reference to formal studies we have performed using the Regenstrief Medical Record (RMR) System at Indiana University Medical Center.[2] In 1972 we started the data base with thirty-two patients from a diabetes clinic. At that time, I thought we would finish the medical record in about a year, and then we would get on to the fun things, such as automatic diagnoses and pattern recognition. I was naive. We are still developing the record. We have had some success: more than twenty years later we have data on 800,000 patients, generated from 600,000 ambulatory visits and 50,000 inpatient encounters per year. The total data base includes over eighty million separate observations from three hospitals on the Indiana University Medical Center campus and thirty outreach clinics scattered throughout the city. The RMR contains results of virtually all diagnostic studies, treatments, vital signs, and inpatient/outpatient encounters. It includes results of clinical laboratory tests, nuclear-medicine

procedures, x rays, CAT scans, and all other formal procedures performed in a hospital. It also includes information on all treatments
as well as the full text of the physician's dictation. The computer
has not replaced the paper chart in our institution yet, but it does
contain most of the information needed to care for the patient. The
paper chart is only rarely used; the computer record reduces both
the work required to maintain the chart and the need to access it.
Soon, we hope to discard the paper chart altogether.

Locating and Transporting Information

The practice of medicine is still in the hunting-and-gathering
stage of social evolution. Physicians spend excessive amounts of
time checking on test results, searching for old x-ray reports, track-
ing old records, and contacting other care providers. The computer-
based medical record can solve these logistic problems, advancing
us to the agricultural stage or beyond. We can stay in one place and
harvest the data through a video screen.

To show the logistic benefits of computer-organized patient
data, we studied the effect of providing flowsheets to physicians in
the emergency room (ER). In a randomized trial, we either presented a flow sheet of the patient's data as the patient came in the
ER door or we did not. We assumed the physicians would behave
differently if they had this information in their hands, and they did.
The intervention reduced test costs by about 14 percent: with the
computer flowsheet, internists spent thirty dollars in testing; without it, they spent thirty-five dollars.[3] Among the surgeons, the differences were approximately the same proportions but were not
statistically significant, because fewer tests are ordered for the cuts
and falls treated by surgeons in the ER.

Feedback and Intelligent Analysis

To the degree that patient information is stored in a structured
and coded format, a computer-based record will also be able to re-
act to its medical content, providing feedback control to the care
system. As in any good engineering system, there are many opportunities to regulate the care process based upon information available to the process. Medical students often think of medicine as a
snapshot—they think they will simply examine the patient, reach a
brilliant conclusion, and close the case. In reality, most medicine
aims at managing a patient's illness. This is a continuous control

effort, and having a stream of data available over time is an important input in the refining of the care process.

The computer record can examine itself and provide reminders and warnings to care providers based upon a set of rules. We assumed that physicians make errors primarily due to oversights— failures to execute rather than failures of knowledge. Errors are inevitable—a natural part of life—and there are a number of psychological studies showing that more errors are made in very busy environments.[4] We assumed that we could reduce the error rates and oversights by having the computer look at the medical record and generate reminders. So we wrote programs to analyze every patient record, using more than 1,400 rules.

We then studied the effect of these computer-generated reminders on physicians' behavior.[5] Over a two-year period, physicians were randomly assigned to either receive these reminders or not; approximately 150,000 reminders were delivered. There were a total of 150 different reminders the computer could suggest. In one study, which produced reminders for residents, faculty, and nurse clinicians, the computer had very significant effects on outcomes. The differences between study and control are quite large, in some cases up to 400 percent, and in each case these differences are statistically significant. What Samuel Johnson said a long time ago, "Man more often needs to be reminded than informed," is still true today. Other have found similar results.[6]

As an aside, we noticed that sociology is as influential as is science in some medical decisions. For example, in 1978 the use of mammography was almost vanishingly small—it was being ordered only 2 percent of the time that it would be appropriate. With the reminders, this increased to 8 percent. We then asked physicians why they weren't ordering mammograms; hadn't they read the American Cancer Society advisories? They gave us two kinds of reasons, one of which was because "no one else does them"; and that was certainly true. The second reason was that they had vague negative attitudes about anything involving radiation.

Up to that point, we had not required physicians to use terminals. They could (and did) use them to retrieve patient data, but they did not have to enter any patient data using the terminals. We then became braver; we put physicians in front of terminals in the outpatient service and asked them to order all their lab tests through the computer. We would perform various interventions as they were ordering tests in the clinic, relaying information on diagnostic efficiency or cost. These interventions reduced test orders in the study group by 9 to 15 percent.[7]

We then got very, very brave and asked the same physicians on the inpatient service to order *everything* on the inpatient service—tests, drugs, diets, nursing orders, etc.—through the computer. I say we were brave because this was not something that physicians had in the past cheerfully accepted. When we developed the PC workstation for the physicians, we included three basic functions: general textbook information, the patient's medical record, and positive and active guidance. We also provided less serious services to reduce computer phobia: computer animated cartoons and satellite weather photos. The main influence we provided was the feedback we gave to the providers as they entered orders. We furnished menus that offered the most effective way to work on or treat a given problem. We provided counterdetailing (supplied messages that countered the hype applied to some expensive drugs). We displayed the prices of everything the physicians ordered in an attempt to raise their cost-consciousness.

We randomly assigned physicians either to use the computer or to use standard paper methods to write orders; we then measured the difference in the cost of care between the cases of the physicians who wrote orders with and without the computer. The effects of this study were significant.[8] Costs were 13 percent lower in the study group compared to the control figures, and length of hospital stay was nearly a day shorter.

Examining Outcomes Across Entire Populations
The computer-based record can also help us to look at the whole picture. When we have access to all the data, from all the patients, we will be able to see patterns in that data that will likely lead to the discovery of clinical truths and the better management of the whole process of care. We can ask: What are really the good outcomes? How does the care process relate to outcomes? What technologies should we invest in? An inkling of the possibilities comes from the Medicare database. Surgical death rates that are reported in the literature as being from 0.5 to 1.0 percent are related as being three to four times higher in the Medicare death data.[9] If this is correct, surgeons should raise their decision thresholds and do fewer of these procedures. Such insights could radically change medical practice in the United States.

The use of large databases (and the inferential statistics required to analyze them) is unfamiliar to most medical researchers. Some argue that you must do a controlled trial to learn anything; but this is not universally true. It is certainly not true in astronomy, where scientists depend solely on observational data—there is a lot of it, and it is often very disordered. Astronomers have invented very sophisticated methods for trading quantity for quality in data. For example, by using special methods for analyzing data—such as spectral power analysis, least squares, nonlinear regression, and specially tailored subroutines—they are able to see things they could not otherwise see. I look forward to the day when statistical methods will have matured to the point that they can provide the same insights from large medical records databases.[10]

We have seen what computers and medical records can do to benefit us. What can we do for them? Large and fairly immediate opportunities exist for reaping the benefits of computer-stored records if we will take advantage of the wealth of patient information that is already stored in computers by health care providers. We find computers everywhere within the health care system. Most of them contain rich amounts of clinical data, but it is scattered across many computer islands (laboratory, billing, pharmacy, automatic EKG carts) within many institutions (nursing homes, community pharmacies, hospitals). If we are to reap the benefits of computer-stored records systems, we need standards for representing all this information electronically so that it can be combined to become a communitywide medical-record system. It would then be possible both to perform statistical analyses and to supply the information to care providers. In particular, we need standards for *codes* that represent tests, procedures, and diagnoses; standards for the structure of the *messages* that carry this information from computer to computer; and standards for *identifying* patients and providers[11] (see Chapter 16).

Opportunities to establish many of these standards already exist in important sectors of the health care industry. If we are to have any hope of achieving these benefits in the near term, we must begin with what exists. A proposal for moving quickly to a first-phase set of standards is being developed by the American Medical Informatics Association (AMIA).[12] We need to settle on the standard identifiers to use for patients, providers, and institutions. In many domains, message standards already exist, and these should be made the message standard for near-term, medical-record data transmission. There are a variety of coding systems that can be patched together to make a fairly complete coding system. We should adopt, in many of these areas, the existing code systems and encourage the federal government to allow the National Library of Medicine (NLM) to build these into a more extensive coding system. By such actions, we will have the messages, codes, and identifiers to rapidly move to the benefits of a computer-stored medical-record system.

Acknowledgment
The research described was supported in part by a grant (Number HS05626) from the Agency for Health Care Policy and Research.

Discussion
In response to an inquiry about reducing paperwork and forms and the possible legal implications of computer-assisted record systems, Dr. McDonald said, "It is clear that being alive can get you sued. But there is some evidence that the risks are less with a computer system utilizing reminders than without." He said there is at least one hospital-information system which has received a reduced malpractice rate because there are certain reminders in the system, thereby reducing the potential for diagnostic or treatment error.

There was a reference to the importance of cartoons or icons to minimize the activation energy barrier often associated with the human/computer interface. There was also a question as to the importance of the Gore Initiative and the national information infrastructure as it related to the medical patient record. McDonald remarked that the large regional or national utilization of medical patient records certainly requires a national information infrastructure. Access to and the use of such an infrastructure has to be somewhat transparent to the local user. Such a national initiative will require the rapid adoption of appropriate standards.

The issue was raised of the confidentiality of individual patient records and the possible resistance of individual medical practitioners to the perusal of their patients' records. It may be that the inclusion of records into a national system might well begin with major hospitals, HMOs, and large group practices, and then later expand to other sectors of the medical health care community. Dr.

McDonald noted that there is a critical mass problem: "Once most are connected, then everyone will want in." Although the confidentiality issue can be used as a weapon to stop such integration, it is likely to evaporate once the process gets started, confidence in mechanisms for protecting confidentiality builds, and the benefits become apparent.

References
1. R.S. Dick and E.B. Steen, eds., *The Computer-Based Patient Record: An Essential Technology for Health Care* (Washington, D.C.: National Academy Press, 1991).

2. C.J. McDonald, W.M. Tierney, J.M. Overhage, D.K. Martin, and G.A. Wilson, "The Regenstrief Medical Record System: 20 Years of Experience in Hospitals, Clinics and Neighborhood Health Centers," *MD Computing* 9(1992): 206–17.

3. G.A. Wilson, C.J. McDonald, and G.P. McCabe, "The effect of immediate access to a computerized medical record on physician test ordering: a controlled clinical trial in the emergency room," *American Journal of Public Health* 72(1982): 698–702.

4. B.L. Drinkwater, "Performance of civil aviation pilots under conditions of sensory input overload," *Aerospace Medicine* 38(1967): 164–68.

5. C.J. McDonald, S.L. Hui, D.M. Smith, W.M. Tierney, S.J. Cohen, and M. Weinberger, "Reminders to physicians from an introspective computer medical record: a two-year randomized trial," *Annals of Internal Medicine* 100(1984): 130–38.

6. C.O. Barnett, R.N. Winickoff, J.L. Dorsey, M.M. Morgan, and R.D. Zielstorff, "A computer-based monitoring system for follow-up of elevated blood pressure," *Medical Care* 21(1983): 400–409.

C.O. Barnett, R.N. Winickoff, J.L. Dorsey, M.M. Morgan, and R.S. Lurie, "Quality assurance through automated monitoring and concurrent feedback using a computer-based medical information system," *Medical Care* 16(1978): 1962–70.

D.C. Classen, S.L. Pestotick, R.S. Evans, and J.P. Burke, "Computerized surveillance of adverse drug events in hospital patients," *Journal of the American Medical Association* 266(1991): 2847–51.

R.M. Gardner, T.P. Clemmer, K.G. Larsen, and D.S. Lohnson, "Computerized alert system used in clinical medicine," *Proceedings of the 32nd Annual Conference on Engineering in Medicine and Biology* (October 1979).

R.K. Hulse, S.J. Clark, C.J. Jackson, H.R. Warner, and R.M. Gardner "Computerized medication monitoring system/protocols," *American Journal of Hospital Pharmacy* 33(1974): 1061–64.

S.J. McPhee, J.A. Bird, D. Fordham, J.E. Rodnick, and E.H. Osborn, "Promoting cancer prevention activities by primary care physicians: results of a randomized, controlled trial," *Journal of the American Medical Association* 266(1991): 538–44.

7. W.M. Tierney, C.J. McDonald, S.L. Hui, and D.K. Martin, "Computer predictions of abnormal test results: effects on outpatient testing," *Journal of the American Medical Association* 259(1988): 1194–98.

W.M. Tierney, C.J. McDonald, D.K. Martin, and M.P. Rogers, "Computerized display of past test results: effect on outpatient testing," *Annals of Internal Medicine* 107(1987): 569–74; and W.M. Tierney, M.E. Miller, and C.J. McDonald, "The effect of test ordering of informing physicians of the charges for outpatient diagnostic tests," *New England Journal of Medicine* 332(1990): 1499–1504.

8. W.M. Tierney, M.E. Miller, J.M. Overhage, and C.J. McDonald, "Physician inpatient order writing on microcomputer workstations," *Journal of the American Medical Association* 269(1993): 379–83.

9. C.J. McDonald and J.K. Fitzgerald, "CABG surgical mortality in different centers," *Journal of the American Medical Association* 267(1992): 932–33.

10. C.J. McDonald and S.L. Sui, "The analysis of humongous databases: problems and promises," *Statistical Medicine* 10(1991): 511–18.

11. C.J. McDonald, D.K. Martin, and J.M. Overhage, "Standards for the electronic transfer of clinical data: progress and promises," *Topics in Health Record Management* 11(1991): 1–16; and C.J. McDonald, "Radiographs by computer for clinicians," *MD Computing* 10(1993): 151–53.

12. The American Medical Informatics Association, 4915 St. Elmo Avenue, Suite 302, Bethesda, MD 20814.

CHAPTER 16

New Strategies for Medical-Imaging Technology

RICHARD I. KITNEY
Imperial College of Science, Technology and Medicine
and
C. FORBES DEWEY
Massachusetts Institute of Technology

"We have recently established an international consortium for medical imaging technology (ICMIT). The aim of the ICMIT program is to change the current pattern of acquisition, diagnosis, retrieval, and storage of images in such a way that the diagnostic process is much more cost-effective."

"Bringing these various image modalities into a common information framework is a key objective."

"Medical equipment manufacturers have tended to adopt a closed architecture approach. Equipment manufacturers must recognize the need for open architecture in equipment design."

To control the costs of diagnostic imaging, it is necessary to examine the technology, the clinical practice, and the modalities of use with the objective of identifying administrative and technological opportunities for improving delivery efficiency and for reducing costs. It is the premise of our program that the only way to be successful in this endeavor is to maintain a global perspective that takes full advantage of modern electronic and computer technology and seeks to gain acceptance for standards and for new methods of diagnostic information delivery.

Open- and Closed-Loop Healthcare Systems
OPEN-LOOP SYSTEMS

The key areas of health care which must be addressed under any advanced health care system are:

- screening,
- prevention,
- diagnosis, and
- treatment.

In many current health care systems these features are not integrated into an overall system. Such systems can be thought of as comprising a single loop, where the patient passes through diagnosis to treatment (Figure 1).

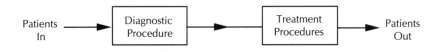

Figure 1. A Traditional Health Care System.

A typical scenario is that the patient visits the hospital and undergoes some form of diagnostic scan, such as a simple chest x ray. The clinician may not see the patient again. The physician's clinical decision may be made on the basis of images and diagnoses passed to him by, say, a radiologist. Patients requiring more than one type of scan are often moved from one department to another. The scan information and associated data is typically stored on hard copy data forms. The information is put in an envelope which is sent to the examining clinician. Long-term storage of the information often involves dividing the information and returning it to its original department. Frequently information either is lost or is sufficiently difficult to retrieve that new tests are performed. If the patient changes his or her health care provider, the records may or may not follow.

The "integration" of information is therefore often done manually by a single clinician studying the data and information on paper and/or film. This exercise is purely for the purposes of clinical diagnosis and does not relate to any form of accounting, either in terms of overall patient statistics or the accounting of resources.

CLOSED-LOOP SYSTEMS

In a closed-loop health care system, patient statistics are monitored for the purposes of determining the system dynamic, that is, the operation of each section of the system. The original open-loop health care system (which could, for example, be a single medical department) is now embedded in an overall closed-loop system comprising several sections (Figure 2). There are two inner loops relating to diagnosis and treatment. Each loop has the same characteristics and consists of a feedback loop of patient/diagnostic statistics. This feeds into a decision dynamic which is partially controlled by the main decision dynamic. The output of the local decision point controls the resource dynamic for the diagnostic loop and the treatment loops, respectively. The input to the local decision dynamic will typically be the number of patients to be treated over a given period. This in conjunction with the local diagnostic information will control the local resource dynamic.

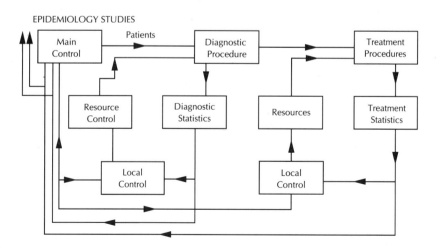

Figure 2. A Module in a Closed-Loop Health Care System. (Note the inclusion of resource control and statistical monitoring.)

We have recently established an international consortium for medical imaging technology (ICMIT). The aim of the ICMIT program is to change the current pattern of acquisition, diagnosis, retrieval, and storage of images in such a way that the diagnostic process is much more cost-effective. A key factor to understand is that there is no reason why the image acquisition process and the diagnostic functions must necessarily be performed in the same physical location. Although data acquisition requires the presence of the patient, it is possible to acquire all the diagnostic information at a site close to the patient's home and then transfer it to the diagnosing clinician, who may be in a totally different part of the country or even in a different country.

The integration and transmission of such information almost by definition requires an electronic medium. Once data in the form of written text, spoken diagnosis, waveforms, images, etc., is stored electronically, full integration of the patient records can be achieved. Transmission nationally or internationally becomes possible. A key aim of the program is to ensure that all generations of computers and scanners can be attached to the system. Once this has been achieved, it will also be possible to uniquely identify each image with an international code which allows secure integration of information from databases at a number of sites.

Medical Image Acquisition and Storage

The processing and analysis of images from various measurement technologies is a major area of growth in the health care sector. Imaging procedures are currently carried out in a wide range of medical specialties, including radiology, cardiology, pediatrics, oncology, neurology, obstetrics, and gynecology.

The rapid development of medical imaging techniques during the last decade has witnessed the emergence and maturation of several new imaging modalities—x-ray-computed tomography (CT), magnetic resonance imaging (MRI), positron emission tomography (PET)—in addition to a significant enhancement of the capability of existing modalities such as conventional x radiography and ultrasound imaging. These new modalities along with developments in the established modalities, such as digital subtraction angiography (DSA), rely heavily on digital-processing techniques. Digitized signals are amenable to a wide range of sophisticated image-restoration and processing methods.

The concept which underlies many of these developments is

that of the picture archival and communication systems (PACS), an all-digital or "filmless" medical-imaging environment. Images are compared and processed on a single imaging workstation, allowing the clinician to view images of a single anatomical site obtained from different modalities. The system will automatically follow a given analysis protocol, which has special features for a given modality, without direct operator involvement.

An extension of the PACS approach is the development of software for 3-D (three-dimensional) modeling of anatomical structures. Such software allows anatomical structures which have been imaged in terms of a series of 2-D slices to be converted into a full 3-D volumetric representation. The slices may be of different image planes through the structure. An exciting aspect of the software is that 3-D solid computer models can be resliced at any orientation and converted back into a series of 2-D images. This facility is seen as being particularly important, because it allows the clinician to cycle between 2-D and 3-D representations of a given structure.

One of the most important trends in medicine today is the attempt to make both diagnostic and therapeutic procedures less invasive. In therapeutics, catheter-tip cameras are used to facilitate keyhole surgery. The treatment of diseased arteries using balloon angioplasty could not be accomplished without simultaneous x-ray angiography. In treatment planning, CT, MR, PET, and nuclear images can give a noninvasive view of human pathology without surgery or other invasive techniques. In monitoring the outcome of therapeutic intervention, the comparison of sequential images is invaluable. Bringing these various image modalities into a common information framework is a key objective of this program.

Key Areas of Technology

Rapid developments in technology are affecting all phases of medical image acquisition and storage. In developing a strategy for the future, it is necessary to identify those areas where change will continue to occur. It will then be possible to design systems capable of handling those future developments as well as current requirements. The areas where change is expected to be especially rapid are:

- computer-imaging processing,
- data storage,
- transmission and retrieval, and
- integration of data from multiple imaging modalities.

Computer processing. The three principal types of scanners in use today are computed tomography (CT), magnetic resonance (MR), and ultrasound. In all three modalities there has been a trend towards the introduction of digital image manipulation. The next stage in this process will be an ever-greater degree of image analysis and processing. To date this often has been carried out by dedicated proprietary systems (usually composed of heavily modified personal computer technology with proprietary electronics), which are used as an adjunct to the main scanner. However, in the future it is likely that such processing will be performed by integrated workstation technology which employs one or more machines across a computer network. Transparent network software operating on computer systems conforming to international standards for open systems is a key technology for the future.

Data storage and retrieval. Until recently, data storage in relation to medical devices was either achieved by making a hard copy or by storing images on analog video cassette tape. In the latter case, the resulting image is usually of much poorer quality than the original. In addition, it is very hard to select an exact sequence, making further manipulation of the images difficult. The use of computer processing enables much more sophisticated forms of data storage and retrieval to be employed. Raw data can be stored in digital form on an optical disk; retrieval is both accurate and rapid. Key issues for the future include image compression, image-transmission methods across a local area or wide area network (LAN or WAN), and intelligent database technology that supports multimedia records.

Integration of data. Medical diagnosis is, by its very nature, a multimodal process. The primary-care physician must use data from a wide variety of sources, including simple data such as personal observations of the patient's health, anecdotal information furnished by the patient, and the patient's pulse rate and blood pressure. To these we now add imaging modalities. In most cases, the data from these different modalities is complimentary and can be used most effectively in combination. CT scans based on x-ray technology provide excellent views of bone structure, while MR images reveal detail about soft tissue. Proper digital integration of these imaging techniques can lead to a composite view of the pathology that is not available from individual measurements.

The very act of bringing all the related records into a consistent format, available to the examining physician at the geographical decision point, will be in itself a major contribution to diagnostic efficiency. The hard-copy folder which is crammed with records of disparate form and uncertain origin make finding and collating diagnostic data very difficult. Because records from many imaging modalities are stored separately, the records frequently cannot be brought to the examination in a timely fashion. Key technological issues that must be addressed are the data base technology supporting the multimedia records and user interface technology that gives the physician easy access to the stored data.

Conclusion. In order to develop a new strategy for local or wide area medical-imaging environments, it is important to define a medical-imaging space comprising applications, technologies, and modalities (Figure 3). Past and current strategy in the design of

THE MEDICAL IMAGING SPACE

Modalities

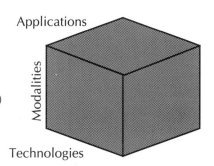

Ultrasound
X-Ray
Computed Tomography (CT)
Magnetic Resonance (MR)
Positron Emission Tomography (PET)
Nuclear Imaging
Electrocardiogram
Microscopy
Chromatography

Applications

Orthopedics
Cardiology
Oncology
Histology
Pathology
Surgery
Obstetrics
Gynecology
Neurology
Nephrology
Pulmonary

Technologies

Computer Hardware
Scanner Equipment
Computer Software
Data Transmission
Data Storage
Data Compression
Databases
Visualization
Multi-Media
Expert Systems
Neural Networks

Figure 3. The Medical-imaging Space, including Applications, Technologies, and Modalities.

medical-imaging technology has been to develop techniques and devices which are both application- and modality-specific. For example, the image-processing and data-storage methods used in a particular magnetic resonance scanner are likely to be unique to scanners from a particular manufacturer and not easily transferable to a remote viewing console. It is very difficult to transport images, data, etc., between a given MR scanner and a remote viewing console developed by another manufacturer, because medical equipment manufacturers have tended to adopt a closed-architecture approach and no hierarchical-imaging strategy has been developed which allows image analysis and data processing to become both modality- and application-independent.

We shall now develop such a strategy.

New Strategies for the Wide Area Imaging Environment

In order to develop strategies powerful enough to encompass both current and future requirements in diagnostic imaging, it is necessary to understand the different segments of the process. These segments relate to the acquisition, compression, storage, transmission, manipulation, and cross-modality correlation of image data. This strategy represents the integrating principles behind a wide—possibly worldwide—radical imaging network which we call MEDINET.

Components of the imaging process: MEDINET will require the development of a structured data-processing environment that serves all four levels of the medical diagnostic hierarchy. It will be necessary to connect a wide range of scanners and other information systems to the network. If the network is to be effective, it will have to cope with a number of generations of equipment which have been developed by different manufacturers over many years. Data will have to be stored, moved around the network, and integrated with data, text, and images from other devices.

Level 1 is concerned with the acquisition and storage of data from a large range of medical devices, some of which present data in analog form. It will be essential to define specific guidelines, and often software and hardware, for analog-to-digital conversion. In the case of a scanner which already provides data and images in digital form, it will be necessary to develop interfacing software, running on a suitable platform, to allow access to the network. This process will also involve the optimization of the images from each modality feeding the integrated system. It will require the development of processing schemes which are specific to the exact nature of the modality in question and which, ideally, are based on a detailed knowledge of the imaging process.

Level 2 activities are concerned with the storage, transfer, and display of all image types on MEDINET. This requires detailed consideration of the optimum coding and compression schemes appropriate to the various images (with careful attention to the maintenance of diagnostic fidelity). Thus, data or images acquired according to the protocol of Level 1 will be compressed and stored or transmitted by software under Level 2. The software will provide a standard header format ensuring that each image, or data file, can be uniquely identified. The header will contain full information on equipment type, acquisition parameters, and any other processing which has been carried out.

Level 3 relates to the manipulation and integration of data from a wide variety of sources. At the simplest level, this involves processing a single signal or image—for example, a blood-pressure waveform or MR image. Hence, Level 3 activities encompass a variety of signal- and image-processing operations including one-dimensional filtering and spectral estimation; spatial filtering, including edge detection; and textural analysis. The next degree of sophistication comprises integration of images, waveforms, and text for the purpose of producing a medical report. This process will often involve the retrieval of data and images from different databases on a network. In the most extreme case, information may be obtained from a number of sites in different countries. Efficient integration and interpretation of diagnostic data stored as digital records requires a graphical display interface between the physician and the computer. This interface must be easy to operate, support different imaging modalities in a consistent manner, and be flexible enough to accommodate future analysis software.

Level 4 involves the use of computer processing and digital data storage and retrieval, which allows the possibility of integrating image information from more than one modality. One example might be the integration of bone images from a CT scanner with the associated muscle and nerve images obtained from an MR scanner. Such integration has major potential clinical benefits because of the special diagnostic properties of each type of scanner. Once image processing at this level has been completed, it may be necessary to revert to Level 3 in order to store or incorporate the results into a clinical report.

Synthesis of the imaging process: Any successful imaging strategy that serves all of the diagnostic segments of MEDINET described above will need to have certain integrating features:

- It must be capable of accommodating existing standards, such as the American College of Radiology-North American Equipment Manufacturers Association (ACR-NEMA) image header standard, and industry standard database technology existing in the medical community.

- The technology must rest on established worldwide open-system standards for computers. This is absolutely essential in order to reduce the expensive reliance on proprietary systems and captive proprietary technologies. It is also the key that will allow a wide spectrum of the scientific community to contribute imaging technology that will improve diagnostic capabilities and advance image-analysis methods. With open-systems standards, contributions can be made independently, at any of the four segments of the imaging process, without a major restructuring of the other levels being required. It also invites the addition of potentially cost-effective technologies such as expert systems and structured diagnostic techniques.

- The technology must respect and take advantage of the "object nature" of images; they are compound entities with information content that goes far beyond the raw data provided by scanner hardware. A raw image is of little use without an accompanying detailed interpretation of what it is or without the background information about the patient and the circumstances surrounding the image acquisition. It is crucial to successful integration of the individual segments to develop these object-oriented representations. The data processing environment must accommodate a natural evolution of object-oriented technology, which, in its own right, has the capability to provide significant productivity gains in several areas of health care.

- A synthesis of the four levels of MEDINET requires that solutions at each level must anticipate and be consistent with revolutionary changes in any of the key component technologies. In the 1990s it is certain that networks of desktop computers costing no more than current personal computers will possess computational capabilities exceeding 1,000 Mflops. It is possible that advances in superconducting magnet technology will reduce hardware and operating costs of MR scanners to the point that machine amortization and maintenance costs are secondary to the costs of clinical diagnostic time and archival storage.

Details of the Imaging Process

Level 1—Data Acquisition. Within the context of the local area or wide area medical-imaging environment, data acquisition is the first stage in the process of transferring data from a particular type of scanner to the network and then to various computer systems for display and further analysis. In the case of MR and CT scanners, individual manufacturers adopt different standards for data formatting. Indeed, within an individual manufacturer's range of scanners there may be significant differences in data format between current machines, and there certainly are between different generations of machines. There have been numerous attempts to overcome this problem by defining standards for data formatting under different conditions. Such standards will be discussed later. A well-known standard of this type is that proposed by ACR-NEMA.

While the definition of such standards is important and worthwhile, there is a major problem associated with their use. In order for a given standard to work on all the scanners, it is necessary for computers and associated equipment to be designed to conform to the standard. While this may happen in time, at present the large installed base of scanners of different types and modalities do not conform. There also are at least three other significant problems which must be overcome for a standard such as ACR-NEMA to be universally adopted:

- Technology is developing at such a rate that the time scale for the development and adoption of any standard may always be too long.
- Corporate strategies may restrict a given company from complying. For example, if a company is to comply with a universal standard, it must believe in an open-architecture approach in which its scanners and equipment are designed to interface with the equipment of other manufacturers. At least one major manufacturer of medical equipment presently does not believe in this strategy. Its current policy is that within a given hospital all the imaging equipment and computers should be manufactured by a single company.

This is a strategy which is very familiar to the computer hardware world, and it is one that is designed to secure a very significant market share for a single company.

- Groups such as the American College of Radiology are mainly interested in defining standards for a given medical specialty. Further, for a standard to be accepted internationally, it must be compatible with similar standards defined by other equivalent bodies and by the equivalent groups within other specialties.

How can the problem of the incompatibility of data be overcome? By the use of "Superset Technology" in conjunction with the use of a hierarchical-network approach.

Level 2—Data Compression, Storage, and Transmission. A wide range of *data compression* techniques will be available under Level-2 processing. These will include both nonreversible and reversible algorithms such as run-length coding, techniques based on linear estimation, and wavelets.

To date, the *storage of data* and information has mainly been achieved by the use of paper or film. There have been some attempts to electronically store data, particularly standard radiological images like chest x rays. However, in the new strategies for health care it will be necessary not only to store data electronically but also to extract and integrate information from a number of sources. These sources may be the databases of different departments within a single hospital; in the future it will be necessary to integrate information from a number of remote sites. It is important to understand that such information is likely to be of three different types:

- Text data, including patient details (name, age, address, etc.); histories of previous illnesses and investigations; and other general information.
- Signal information, including ECG traces, EMG traces, blood pressure and respiratory waveforms.
- Image information, including x-ray scans, MR and CT scans, etc.

Such information will be required at the time of a particular medical examination and may have to be accessed from a number of remote sites and then integrated. This approach implies the use of multimedia. It is important to note that one key difference between the traditional methods of acquiring data and that of using electronic media is that with the latter the information in the original database is left unchanged. In the case of information stored in the form of hardcopy, the primary information is often removed.

The first step in the retrieval of data is the identification of the data source. In the future it is likely that this will be facilitated by the use of some form of patient information card. In its simplest form, the card would contain basic information such as name, address, date of birth, etc., together with information about where the patient is registered—that is, the location of their primary database. There may be three basic tiers to the hierarchy: a national register, a regional or state register, and a local register. Each patient on the network will have a master index at a local register—either at his/her primary health care center or at a local hospital.

Consider the case of a clinical problem arising while a patient is abroad and the hospital to which he or she is admitted is on an international network. Access to the patient's primary database could be achieved by the use of his/her personal information card. In its most basic form, the required data could be a series of numbers very similar to a telephone number, comprising the country code, area code, and local number. All the information could then be automatically accessed and transported across the network to the clinical decision point. The system would then assemble it in integrated form on the investigating clinician's computer screen.

Object Description

The types of information that can be accessed differ in a number of ways. The basic approach to the access of information must therefore be one that considers each piece of information via an object-oriented approach. Objects may comprise an ECG, blood pressure records, a chest x ray, or an MR image. Clearly, the nature of each of these objects will be very different. Two important considerations are the amount of data comprising each object and the format of the data. There is vast variation in the amount of data arising from different types of objects; the system must be able to accommodate each type as individual objects. The overall formatting of objects is of critical importance in allowing data, signals, and images to be passed across local or wide area networks.

A good example of a modern standard is the new ACR-NEMA standard Digital Imaging and Communications in Medicine (DICOM) version three. It is anticipated that the standard will be available for general use in the first quarter of 1994. The objective of the DICOM development group was to provide a health care system standard which will be capable of encompassing various imaging modalities and medical specialties. It is very important that the information conveyed be specified unambiguously and related to other objects as described above. DICOM image objects are being designed for various types of images, such as MR, CT, PET, ultrasound, and conventional x ray. In addition, the aim is for the standard to be able to transport physiological signals and associated analytical data such as graphs, histograms, statistics, and others.

A second important area which is being addressed by the DICOM standard is networking. The aim is to fully support networking via the TCP/IP and OSI standards. Because the basis of the standard is an object-oriented approach, future developments of the standard should be far more straightforward.

While standards such as DICOM are probably essential, it is nevertheless important to understand that, almost by definition, they are based on a top-down approach strategy, which means that manufacturers of medical equipment are expected to conform to the standard in their new designs. Such standards will not work for systems already installed and for those new systems which do not comply. There are three major problems associated with the adoption of imaging standards such as ACR-NEMA or DICOM.

- The time scale for the development and adoption of a standard may be too long to be of practical use because of the rate at which technology is developing.
- For various strategic reasons major manufacturers may not want an open-architecture approach to be adopted.
- There is likely to be some incompatibility in standards between individual medical specialties and in different countries.

How can these difficulties be overcome? By a three-component strategy:

- a bottom-up approach;
- a hierarchical approach to the local and wide area imaging environments (of which the network is an integral part);
- by the adoption by manufacturers of open architectures.

A key part of the ICMIT strategy is to adopt a bottom-up approach—software will be developed which allows any existing scanner to be interfaced to the network, regardless of whether it complies to a standard like ACR-NEMA. This is what we call Superset Technology (Figure 4). Taking the example of a generic scanner, data from the scanner passes through a translator which converts the data to a form that can be transmitted across the network. The remote computer which is receiving the data has, as its first stage of processing, a second translator, which converts the data to a form that is capable of being read by the computer's user interface. The superset software within the translator provides a "wrapper" within which all the information relating to the object being transferred is stored—i.e., data format, standard information (e.g., from the ACR-NEMA standard), type of image, etc.

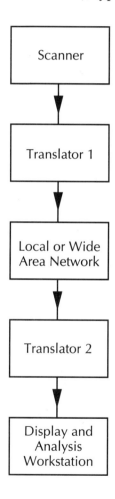

Figure 4. Superset Technology—the ICMIT Bottom-Up Approach to Interface *Any* Existing Scanner to the Network.

The adoption of this approach means that at the first stage (Level 1), the data object is detached from its hardware source and becomes an independent entity on the network. Once the data object has passed through the translator associated with the scanner, it becomes hardware independent. This is very important because other medical network strategies are based on the concept of the "remote computer" accessing the scanner directly, taking the data in raw form across the network and carrying out all the processing steps at the remote computer—which implies that the operator of the remote computer has to have information about every scanner on the network.

Level 3—Data Manipulation and Integration. The third level of the hierarchical medical-imaging environment comprises the processing of images and data. At this level, analysis is modality independent. (Level 2 of the system, operating under the Flexfile format, will automatically compensate for the characteristics of the modality). Hence, the system operator (e.g., the examining clinician) will be aware of the modality from which a particular image originates (together with other basic information), but will be free to process different images using identical mathematical techniques.

Level 4—Cross Modality Data Integration. Level 4 is the highest level of the imaging system. Under this level, the system operator has the ability to process images from more than one modality, using identical mathematical techniques, including arithmetic operations such as the summation of whole images.

Conclusions

We have discussed some of the ways in which modern medical-imaging technology can be applied to a range of data. The data may have originated from groups working in various medical specialties; been recorded on scanners operating under different modalities; and/or been transported across a telecommunications network to a remote viewing station, typically comprising a standard workstation. It is our view that the effective implementation of local and wide area medical-imaging networks requires the application of two key criteria:

- equipment manufacturers must recognize the need for open architecture in equipment design; and
- an effective local area or wide area network must be capable of handling data objects in the form of images, sig-

nals, data, text, etc., with equal efficiency. This will involve the processing and display of such objects in integrated form on a single screen, often at the clinical decision point. Another requirement is that such a system must be capable of accommodating the large range of medical equipment which forms the already installed base at hospitals throughout the world.

Acknowledgment

We acknowledge the support of other members of the ICMIT Consortium in the preparation of this paper.

CHAPTER 17

Discussion: Information and Communication Technology in Radiology

DOUGLAS MAYNARD
Bowman-Gray School of Medicine
Wake Forest University
Winston-Salem, North Carolina

"Information and communication technology is one area in radiology where you can actually improve the care of the patient and at the same time actually reduce costs."

Radiology has been interested in information and communication technology for a long time; the field is very active in developing programs with industry and government. Our department designed and implemented our own radiology information system (RIS) in the 1970s because there wasn't one available at that time. In the last ten years we have collaborated with Bell Laboratories to develop what we call "filmless radiology." We feel that information and communication technology is one area in radiology where you can actually improve the care of the patient and at the same time actually reduce costs. There is technology currently available that can be readily applied; we need to see how it can work in the health field to improve care and decrease costs.

We have worked in the areas of telemedicine, teleradiography, and high-speed networks. There are two areas which illustrate the potential. First, we have integrated our hospital information system, RIS, and our images and digital voice system. What does this do for us? From a patient care standpoint, when a patient gets admitted to the hospital or outpatient facility, the patient is given a hospital unit number, a name, a location, and a position—that information then tracks that patient throughout the entire hospital and throughout the radiology department. What this means is that we have much more adequate data from a patient-care standpoint. Some of the information in the computer allows us to determine if a test is being done appropriately for the patient's specific disease or problem. It also allows very quick retrieval of information for the clinician—either in voice, text, or imaging forms. This provides our clinicians with information they can act on quickly. And how does this decrease costs? We have found that a large number of clerical jobs are no longer needed, because we don't have to keep reentering the information. The amount of transcription time has decreased. There are other savings that can't be easily documented, such as travel to and from the x-ray department by clinicians. It has been shown that information that can be immediately transferred from one place to another really does decrease the length of a patient's stay within the hospital.

Second, we have installed a high-speed network connecting all seven buildings in the medical center complex. In conjunction with the General Electric Corporation, we have put in a network with our six CTs and two MRs so that a clinician or physician can actually view the study from any location. How does this improve care? We have an outpatient facility that is about one mile away that we do not staff with a radiologist, but we have technologists there who do twenty to thirty CTs per day. That remote clinic has a fiber-optic link into the main hospital, so the patient can go to a very accessible outpatient facility and have the study done. That patient can be monitored concurrently by the physician or radiologist residing at the main inpatient activity. The patient's images are then transmitted to the main facility to be viewed—either on a screen or printed—and sent to the proper radiologist. If the patient has a head study, for example, it goes to a neuroradiologist. This decreases costs because we are not staffing that facility with a radiologist—we have one who is already on line in the hospital.

There are many possibilities to apply this technology in the future to both improve patient care and to decrease costs. It may only be limited by our imagination of how it can be used.

Discussion

Dr. Donald Detmer, discussion moderator, pointed out that the computer-based patient record report of the Institute of Medicine[1] was a very unique study. It was one of the first studies to be internally commissioned by the Institute of Medicine, because the institute had concluded that the technology was both available and changing rapidly, and that such a study was timely and important. The study pointed out the need for national standards, also addressed by McDonald in Chapter 15. The report advocated the formation of the Computer-based Patient Record Institute (CPRI), which is now in existence, to serve as a public and private focus for the development of standards and technology.

It was pointed out that the proof that a standard is good is that it does the job. TC/PIP was given as an example. There was a reference to the American Standards Institute, which is the U.S. agency that officially communicates with the International Standards Organization (ISO). It was pointed out that there is a committee, the ACR-NEMA Committee, working on standards for the radiology community. The work of the EMLS was also noted.

References

1. R.S. Dick and E.B. Steen, eds., *The Computer-Based Patient Record: An Essential Technology for Health Care* (Washington, D.C.: National Academy Press, 1991).

PART V

•

INNOVATION AND OPPORTUNITIES

•

CHAPTER 18

•

Empowering Patient Decision Making

JOHN WENNBERG
Dartmouth School of Medicine

"We really don't know very much about what patients want in medicine, because we rarely ask them. . . . There is nothing in the clinical history . . . which allows us to predict what patients want. . . . We were operating on people who didn't want surgery."

"How well have we evaluated the impact of these treatments on patients? . . . The answer is—not very well at all."

"The assessment, by the patients, of *their* symptoms is very important, even decisive, with regard to choice of treatment."

"The goal is to give each patient the best available information about his or her particular medical condition, so that the patient can share in the treatment choice with the physician, understanding and expressing his or her personal preferences in certain key areas. That choice has never been presented quite this way."

"This strategy of bringing the patient into the equation may actually lead to a reduction in the use of care."

Copyrighted material © 1994; *Medical and Biological Engineering in the Future of Health Care*, edited by J.D. Andrade; University of Utah Press.

"Physicians always thought that there was too much information presented and the patients wouldn't understand it; whereas the patient groups seemed to agree that the amount of information was about right, and they indeed did understand it. People really can deal with information."

What is the relevance for patients of outcome research? Where are we now in terms of our real understanding of the health care crisis? Much of the rhetoric suggests that progress in biomedical science and technology has reached the point where we no longer can afford what patients want, that we need to ration care. We are *not* at that point. Although we do have new ideas and technologies, we are not at all certain how well all those technologies work for the individual patient or for the patient collective. Moreover, we really don't know very much about what patients want in medicine, because we rarely ask them.

Background

My background is that of an epidemiologist looking at the difference in the rate of surgical procedures and medical-care delivery as a function of where patients live. We found some enormous differences in the risk of surgery depending on where you live. The relative risk of having a bypass operation if you live in New Haven as compared to Boston is two to one—for residents of these communities, not for people who come from outside to have surgery. The probability for a hysterectomy is twice as high for a New Haven woman as it is for a Bostonian. Hip replacements are about 70 percent more frequent in the Boston area, and carotid artery surgery is about 2.2 times more common if you live in Boston. The basic point is not that people in these different communities are being under- or over-treated, but that they are being treated *differently.* The following lists the conditions and their options:

Condition	Treatment Options
Angina	Surgery vs. Angioplasty vs. Drugs vs. Watchful Waiting
Menopausal Bleeding	Surgery vs. Hormones vs. Drugs vs. Watchful Waiting

| Arthritis of the Hip | Surgery vs. Drugs vs Watchful Waiting |
| Threat of Stroke | Surgery vs. Aspirin |

Such data as we found raises the questions: Which rate is right? What works in medicine? What do patients want? How well have we evaluated the impact of these treatments on patients? And the answer to the last question is—not very well at all.

There are rules that require that drugs be evaluated before they reach the market, but we have no rules for reevaluation once a drug is in the market. Drugs can be used for any purpose that the physician may discover. New ways of treatment are often discovered in the context of clinical practice; new options open up. Our own studies of prostate disease showed that drugs approved for hypertension—namely, alpha blockers—became empirically useful in treating the symptoms of prostate disease; but we found this without clinical trials. Generally, surgery doesn't get clinical trials. Not a single clinical trial was done for prostate disease.

We need to articulate a science policy that promotes evaluation. We need a policy for the evaluative sciences as distinct from the biomedical sciences. We have not made that distinction clear. We do have the FDA and the Agency for Health Care Policy and Research; we also have the NIH, which sometimes does clinical trials and sometimes not. We have no orderly process for assuring that the evaluations are done. An exception is patient-outcomes research teams. These interdisciplinary groups of epidemiologists, biostatisticians, clinicians, individuals expert in functional status measures, and others have been given a task of systematically patrolling the problems associated with a particular condition. There is a PORT (patient-outcomes research team) for most of the conditions listed above.

The Prostate

Our group has been interested in the prostate. When we began our research we could see regional variations. For example, in some parts of the state of Maine, 50 percent of men were having their prostates operated on for benign prosthetic hypertrophy by the time they reached 85 years; in other communities, it was less than 10 percent. The option at that time seemed to be benign neglect. As we began to research the situation with surgeons from different parts of the state and began to put together a large database, we learned there were no clinical trials. There was in fact very little information on the theoretical reasons for doing prostate surgery. Some surgeons believe that early surgery helps people live longer because surgery later when people were older and sicker was avoided—a theory of preventive surgery. Others believed the surgery helped the patient feel better—a quality of life philosophy of surgery. By piecing this information together, we were able to demonstrate that there was no likely advantage in terms of life expectancy from early surgery. The disease was not as pernicious in its natural progression as many urologists thought, and if the patient waited and lived with the symptoms, he probably would not develop renal disease, bladder obstruction, or conditions which would require surgery.

It became clear that prostate surgery was a quality of life operation if it was of any value at all. There was no evidence about the actual impact of prostatectomy on men. We could find no single study in the literature that declared how symptoms and quality of life were affected in any systematic way. With this background, we began to develop a more articulate vision of what outcomes research is, as distinct from other types of biomedical research. The metric used to evaluate the result of prostatectomy was urine flow. The assumption was that if you urinated more easily you felt better or lived longer—a typical reductionist-type notion that focuses on one measurable aspect of physiology. What did matter to patients was how they urinated and how they felt. It mattered to them if they could have sex, and it mattered to them if there were risks with the operation. By getting focus groups of patients together and asking them what was at stake, we were able to develop an inventory of what mattered to the patient. It wasn't just symptoms, it was fear of cancer. We found that people were bothered to different degrees by symptoms. Some had very noticeable symptoms but were not worried very much about them. The subjective aspects became important. The assessment, by the patients, of *their* symptoms is very important, even decisive, with regard to choice of treatment.

If a patient chooses surgery for his benign prostate hypertrophy, the probability is that his symptoms will be improved. We did an exhaustive series of studies in which we simply followed up on patients who had surgery. Although we had no controls, there were a few randomized clinical trials of drugs which didn't work too well and gave us a sense of the control population. It was clear from the point of view of symptom improvement that prostate surgery was effective. We also found that there were certain risks associated with the benefits, including incontinence, impotence, and death as a result of the operation.

On the watchful waiting side, the symptoms we discovered from a few natural history studies were quite variable. Some people would get better, some worse, and most stayed the same. But if one chose watchful waiting, one avoided the risks mentioned above—a benefit of watchful waiting—but there was also a greater risk of acute retention.

That ended the second phase of our investigation of the prostate. The first was the discovery of the variability; the second, the questions of what was the theoretical basis of this controversy, why were people doing things differently, and what were the outcomes and theoretical structure of the decision problem. We came to a reasonable conclusion about four or five years ago. We had accumulated a large database that gave us reasonably precise probability estimates for many subgroups of men. By the state of symptoms and operative mortality rates we were able to predict patient conditions and the severity of illness. What became clear was that we had a very large set of probabilities which had to be communicated to patients, because rational choice depends on the patient's information. So, we had a communication problem. One effective way to get information summarized and relevant to a subgroup is to use a computer. You enter in information about the patient characteristics, symptoms status, and disease status, and you get the best estimate that you can for that particular subgroup. Easy to do.

How do you communicate to patients that they have options? Our problem became the melding of the probabilities of outcomes with the value the patient applies to the outcomes. We turned to interactive video technology. We were able to present to patients scenarios of their future depending upon their choices. The problem of how to communicate probabilities to patients became the subject for this part of our research. The interactive video strategy turned out to be useful because of two features:

- we could get the probability correct for the patient's subgroup and get the patient to see scenarios of the future, so he could begin to make his own evaluations; and,
- by virtue of having all that information, we were in a position to do more sophisticated studies than had previously been done. As distinct from a clinical trial where random-

ization is the key feature, we could now undertake a clinical trial in which the preference of the patient became a key
factor in the choice of treatment.

We have been able to follow up large numbers of patients and
to begin to fill in missing probabilities. For example, one of the
most important probabilities to a man who has acute urinary retention and is successfully catheterized, in the sense that he can now
urinate again, is what is the chance that it will happen again. If the
chances are 5 percent or 100 percent, there is a big difference in the
choice. The database that was available would not allow us an accurate estimate, except we were certain from one study in the U.K.
that it was not 100 percent. We think it was about 5 percent, but we
had to tell the patients in our scenario that. We are now beginning
to follow up a number of patients who have elected watchful waiting after that stage, and that probability estimate will now be possible to be updated.

There are two important dimensions of this particular strategy.
The first is communication—to improve the ethical nature and status of the doctor-patient relationship by making it possible and appropriate for the patient to make a choice. The second dimension is
to do longitudinal studies to update and make better use of available information.

The interactive video, "A Shared Decision-Making Program,"
isn't just an educational video. It is designed to give patients the
information they need to *participate* in their medical-treatment decisions. It is called "shared" because it is used in the health care setting, with the doctor referring patients to this clinical information
tool. The topics are medical conditions for which patient preference
is important in choosing among alternative treatments. The goal is
to give each patient the best available information about his or her
particular medical condition so that the patient can share in the
treatment choice with the physician, understanding and expressing
his or her personal preferences in certain key areas. That choice has
never been presented quite this way.

The program is delivered using an interactive video disk. It
looks and feels like a television program, with an important difference: personal information about each user is entered into the computer before each viewing—things like age, symptoms, and test
results. This determines what that person sees; each viewer re-
ceives information tailored to his or her own situation. The benign

prostatic hyperplasia video involves two physicians describing *their* different decisions as BPH patients, one choosing surgery and the other choosing a nonsurgical approach. Viewers are given more detailed information about some of the possible complications. For example, they are told about acute retention, an uncomfortable possible complication of watchful waiting, but one that is not dangerous if treated promptly. A viewer's own probabilities of experiencing the various outcomes are presented to him graphically.

The evaluation process for the BPH program involved more than one thousand patients seeing the program at ten different sites across the U.S., Canada, and the U.K. The response from patients, physicians, nurses, and health care administrators has been overwhelmingly positive.

We have used this program most successfully in prepaid group practices, because the surgeons there are on salary and can readily shift their practice when patient demand changes. The important point here is the distinction between the preferences and attitudes of the patient and the objective situation. There is nothing in the clinical history, physical exam, urine flow, or symptom levels which allows us to be able to predict what patients want. We are learning that their concerns about impotence and the degree of discomfort they have with their symptoms ultimately determine their choice.

After we implemented the interactive video, we found that only one out of five men with severe symptoms chose surgery. The rest chose watchful waiting. The implications are quite clear. If practice guidelines had been set in place to say that patients should be operated on if they have severe symptoms, there wouldn't be a physician in the United States who would have disagreed. Yet it turned out that when patients were asked what they wanted, only one in five actually chose surgery. Retrospectively, it appears that we were operating on people who didn't want surgery.

We asked patients how much they were bothered by their symptoms and how much they were concerned about impotence, since those factors became the desiderata of choice. In the regression studies we did, symptoms no longer even entered the equation after we asked about attitudes in regard to impotence and degree of discomfort. This unveils a new concern and area in medicine that we need to begin to consider.

Patient Preferences

All of the profession's technology has been focused on the notion that the physician is the sole and sufficient agent for making decisions for patients. In many cases, that is quite reasonable. For example, if one has an acute myocardial infarction and there is a preferred algorithm for survival, survival would be everybody's preference. The algorithm works fine. In addition, for some major surgical endeavors there are also preference-based choices for most patients, even in the case where life is extended. In our work now with interactive video disks dealing with cancer, we are finding that women will commonly forego the risks of chemotherapy, accepting a slightly elevated increase of risk of recurrence in order to avoid the downsides of chemotherapy—a perfectly rational choice.

Generally, in the case of BPH, we have found that patients tend to be more risk-averse than their advising physicians. If this is a general reaction, we might expect that the strategy of bringing the patient into the equation may actually lead to a reduction in the use of care. In fact, in the prepaid group practices in which we have been doing these experiments, we have seen declines in surgical rates of about 50 percent, and they were already relatively low in these HMOs as compared with the rest of the country. This brings up interesting questions. If we begin to uncouple supplier-induced demand and we begin to shift what we know and don't know onto the patient, we will clearly end up with a market that has different dimensions and requirements than the market we know now.

The number of urologists available has had nothing to do with these issues. The number of urologists is related to the needs of residency programs and hospitals to staff themselves and has little to do with the demand in the market. The number of urologists employed in the prepaid group practices was in excess of the amount demanded in that setting. When we compare the number of physicians hired by prepaid group practices to the numbers available in the U.S. economy as a whole, we see massive excesses—there are 60 percent more urologists in the rest of the economy than are hired by prepaid group practices and 250 percent more surgeons!

A New Rationale

If we begin to focus on the patient, and if we can develop a strategy of consistent evaluation with the probability estimates for these conditions continually updated, then we have an opportunity to enter a new phase of treatment. As we began our studies, we had

three possibilities: transurethral prostatectomy versus open prostatectomy versus watchful waiting. By 1992 new items were coming
into the market. Balloon dilations are an outgrowth of the success
of angioplasty. An enterprising urologist in Boston figured that if it
works for the coronary artery, why would it not work for the prostate. He formed a small company, developed a balloon, got FDA
approval, and is now marketing it—without clinical evidence of
how it works or compares to other conditions. An alpha-blocker
drug became popular after its introduction by some urologists.
Then along came Proscar, a drug designed to work on the prostate.
Another new idea was hypothermia—you could heat it up, make
it shrink, and help people urinate more easily. Along came another
idea of putting in little tents—again from the medical technology
industry—little tents to shore it up. Another surgical idea is TUIP,
transurethral incisional prostatectomy, an incision of the prostate
rather than the "roto rooter" procedure that is usually associated
with the transurethral prostatectomy. Finally, lasers got to the prostate. So, all these technologies came in, and we have now introduced some of them into the interactive video.

One of the most disappointing aspects of our whole research
project, however, has been the fact that we have not been able to get
funding to do clinical trials on these things—there is no mechanism available for doing clinical trials. Our dilemma now is how to
go the next step—to gain an orderly strategy for evaluation.

Discussion

It was noted that the work presented utilized well-educated
and informed patients. Are there any problems or limitations using
it for the general man or woman on the street? Dr. Wennberg responded that the patient populations involved a broad cross-
section of backgrounds, both educational and racial, including a
Veteran's Administration hospital population. He pointed out that
the physicians always thought that there was too much information
presented and that the patients wouldn't understand it, whereas
the patient groups seemed to agree that the amount of information
was about right, and they indeed did understand it. He said, "I
think people really can deal with information."

It was noted, however, that there is a report in the pediatric literature related to institutional review boards and informed consent
suggesting that more poorly educated individuals tend dispropor-
tionately not to participate—they tended to be more intimidated,

and backed out of research studies. It was mentioned also that there is very little literature on this topic. Another commentator said that consent forms have been targeted to the sixth- to eighth-grade level, but it is clear that they need to be targeted to the first-grade educational level.

It was noted by J. Andrade that an informal evaluation of IRB forms of five different urban hospitals concluded they "were abominably written; they were very difficult to understand at any grade level. I think the problem is writing and communication skills. Physicians are no better at it than engineers. They are both atrocious." There was general agreement.

Reference

1. T. Randall, "Producers of Videodisc Programs Strive to Expand Patient's Role in Medical Decision-Making Process," *Journal of the American Medical Association* 270 (1993): 160–62.

CHAPTER 19

Minimally Invasive Surgery: Big Procedures Through Small Holes

JOHN HUNTER
School of Medicine, Emory University

"When the bar is set too high, the surgeon fails and the patient falls—and then industry is nowhere in sight."

"It was industry pushing new procedures on the public despite a lack of evident benefit. . . . I should have asked them how they spelled *integrity*."

"The potential savings is nearly half a billion dollars. But this isn't the only advantage. The greatest advantage is getting people back to work and to play more rapidly."

"We need to find ways to put our hand back in the abdomen through these little tiny incisions, or ultimately through no incision at all."

I like to think that an associate professor of surgery should be someone strutting around hospital corridors with a pod of residents and students behind him, or someone involved in the OR in theatrical dissections of the living. What I do may be disappointing to you—I watch television all day! The television monitor that I watch provides a two-dimensional image of a tissue I am working on with footlong instruments, six to eight inches beneath the abdominal wall. The image is dependent on a 300-watt light source to illuminate the abdomen, a fiber-optic guide to get the light into the patient, a rigid telescope only one centimeter in diameter to conduct the image out of the patient, a high-resolution video camera perched on the end of the telescope to receive that image, and two video monitors—so that both surgeon and assistant can see what they are doing without getting a stiff neck. This is called laparoscopic surgery, and it is but one small component of minimally invasive surgery. The term "minimally invasive surgery" has been assaulted by some surgical philosophers as being as much of an oxymoron as "somewhat pregnant." "Surgical philosophers" is itself perhaps an oxymoron. The term "minimally invasive surgery" has stuck, however, because the procedures described lie somewhere between noninvasive procedures that do not violate the skin, such as shock-wave fragmentation of kidney stones, and procedures that leave a big gash—traditional hands-on operative therapy.

Minimally invasive surgeries are procedures that were once performed with a large gash and that can now be performed with a small slit or with no incision at all, utilizing natural body orifices such as the mouth. Big procedures through small holes, indeed. At this juncture we should recognize that we surgeons are still one step away from the ideal, which would be truly non-invasive, seamless surgery. Although I recently co-edited the first North American text to try to cover the technologies and techniques of minimally invasive surgery,[1] laparoscopic surgery is what I know best. Developments in laparoscopic abdominal surgery will serve in this paper as a paradigm for minimally invasive surgery. Although my focus is laparoscopic surgery, the story is little different for coronary artery dilatation, arthroscopic surgery of the knee, or any of a dozen procedures practiced by interventional radiologists.

The history of laparoscopic surgery is short. Although individuals have been putting primitive endoscopes through the abdominal wall and down the gullet for a century, modern endoscopic surgery dates back to the early 1960s, at which time flexible, fiberoptic coherent bundles were developed to conduct light around corners. Laparoscopic surgery was made possible with the development of the solid-rod-lens telescope, which transmitted significantly more light than previous air-filled telescopes, allowing adequate illumination of the gas-inflated peritoneum for the first time in history. For twenty years surgeons pressed their eyes to the ends of these telescopes; but they were severely limited in what they could do by the need to hold the endoscope with one hand, leaving only a single hand to perform the surgery. In the late 1980s, laparoscopy went video. The ability to work off a video monitor decreased eyestrain, increased the length of procedures that could be accomplished, and allowed many hands and imaginative minds to become involved in the procedure; it also increased the complexity of the procedures that could be performed. Teaching endoscopy become a joy instead of a trial. It should be no surprise that with the availability of video laparoscopy, groups of surgeons in France, Germany, and the U.S. simultaneously developed the technique of laparoscopic gallbladder removal, also known as laparoscopic cholecystectomy, or lap chole, for short.

Lap chole requires four small punctures—one for the telescope and three others for operating instruments. If lap chole had been a drug or instrument rather than an operation, it would have undergone three phases of testing: a small phase-one study to prove safety, phase two to establish efficacy, and a phase-three prospective randomized trial to prove that it was better than open cholecystectomy. These procedures were not subject to such scientific rigor because the public became the judge—after all, this is a democracy—the public overwhelmingly voted with their feet that they wanted their gallbladders removed with the new laser surgery. It was an accident of history that excitement about laser medicine was peaking at the time lap chole was introduced, offering laser manufacturers the opportunity to sell a laser to every fifty-bed community hospital that hoped to corner the local market on lap chole operations.

This brings me to a story that typifies one of the potential problems with the industrial support of research. When I was at the University of Utah, I was asked to run a prospective randomized trial comparing laser lap chole with electrosurgical lap chole. In order to run this trial, I obtained the support of both a laser company and an electrosurgical company, each providing me the necessary equipment. Halfway through the trial, I ran out of laser fibers and called the laser company to replenish my supply. They asked how the study was going, and I informed them that I hadn't cracked the data yet, but it appeared that the two methods were about equivalent. At this point they said they were going to recall their laser and provide no more fibers; they said, "Why would a laser company want to support a study that wasn't going to show the laser was better?" I suggested to them that they should because they said that they would. That argument didn't seem to phase them. In a calmer moment, I concluded that I should have asked them how they spelled *integrity.*

Other problems that have sprung up in the relationships between surgeons and corporations are conflicts of interest and the premature promotion of new procedures. Conflicts of interest often arise during the education of surgeons in new procedures. The accepted format for educating a practicing surgeon has been a short course over a long weekend, in order not to pull the surgeon away from his or her practice for too long. Course directors, in an effort to keep costs down and remain competitive with industry-sponsored courses, have been forced to rely upon industry to supply equipment for hands-on training. The AMA has approved such activity as long as lectures and printed material are not blatant corporate advertisement. Clearly, however, the presence of one company's product rather than another's at a surgical course is tacit endorsement, and it well may be in conflict with an optimal education. Less-than-ethical arrangements involve sales commissions—also known as kickbacks—offered to surgeons for sales of high-priced items such as lasers to the students attending that surgeon's course. Industry has been very involved in the development of new procedures, pushing more and more procedures by laparoscopy, hoping to have first access to the production of the instruments necessary to perform these procedures. When the procedures have been tested in animals, and the FDA has given its blessing, we have seen the phenomenon of corporations hyping procedures and putting undue pressure on practitioners to try things that the practitioners are not sure is right or in the best interest of their patients. When the bar is set too high, the surgeon fails and the patient falls—and then industry is nowhere in sight.

A case in point is laparoscopic hernia repair, which was recently assailed in an editorial in a leading surgical journal as "the socioeconomic tyranny of surgical technology." I think what they were trying to say is that the corporations supplying hernia equipment were pushing this procedure on the public and on surgeons before it had been adequately evaluated. To be fair, it was not truly surgical technology which was pushing the system, it was industry pushing new procedures on the public despite a lack of evident benefit. The only thing that is clear about laparoscopic hernia repair is that it is more expensive than is open hernia repair. In Seattle, it costs the patient and insurer an average of $1,500 more than hernia repair. In Atlanta, the difference was even more striking—with a $6,200 difference between laparoscopic and open hernia repair.

Compare this with lap chole which costs society $800 *less* than open chole in our study at the University of Utah. If one multiples this by 600,000 cholecystectomies performed each year, the potential savings is nearly a half-billion dollars. But this isn't the only advantage. The greatest advantage is getting people back to work and to play more rapidly. No one has been able to figure out how much money in otherwise lost work time laparoscopic surgery has saved this country, but it should be greater than the procedural savings. Suffice it to say that probably most of you feel that if you were gone from your labs for a week on vacation, things wouldn't suffer too greatly. But if you were gone an unplanned absence of four to six weeks, havoc would result. More importantly, imagine the disaster if our secretaries, lab techs, and nurses were gone for four to six weeks. In general, minimally invasive surgery gets patients back in the work force in a week, while standard surgery requires four to six weeks for the patient to reach the same degree of recovery. Clearly, if performed responsibly, laparoscopic surgery has the ability to save billions of health care dollars.

Industry was critical to the laparoscopic revolution, rapidly providing optics and instruments to meet an incredible, almost instantaneous demand. Without the involvement of private-sector industry in Germany, Japan, and the U.S., we would not be nearly as far along as we are in our ability to perform minimally invasive surgery. Industry has led the way in providing new technology, applying new, compact, color-chip CCD cameras, and more recently providing 3-D imaging. Tasks that many surgeons in 1992 found too difficult using two dimensions such as suturing and knot tying, are more easily performed with 3-D imaging. Yet another challenge, the ability to sew tissue back together after removing the diseased section, may be achievable by the average general surgeon with stereo optics—another development of private-sector industry.

Industry has been a ready source of revenue to do laparoscopic research, but there are strings attached. By its very nature, industrial research is technology driven. The initiative is to test the latest gadget and see what it can do. If it doesn't perform well, the study is suppressed while the instrument is redesigned. Scientific research, in contrast, is hypothesis driven. Technology supplies the means to test the hypothesis, but it is not an end in itself.

Several engineering laboratories are working to produce very interesting microrobots which might be used in minimally invasive surgery. ARPA has interests in virtual-reality surgical simulators (see Chapter 12). In addition to telepresence, robots, and simulators, what are other future directions of minimally invasive surgery? Surgeons, radiologists, gastroenterologists, and others will develop more combined endoscopy/laparoscopy procedures, and engineers will develop more compact instruments. One of the trends we have seen recently is for instrumentation to get larger, requiring larger access ports—I think we are beginning to lose sight of what minimally invasive surgery really is. Most laparoscopic instruments open and close like a hand, but there is no wrist movement involved. Adding articulation to simulate wrist movements would be valuable for more complex surgical tasks. One of the real missing elements of laparoscopic surgery is the loss of tactile sense. Strain gauges have been used to try to replace that tactile sense, but my experience with them suggests that they are still fairly primitive. We need to find ways to "put our hand back" in the abdomen through these little tiny incisions, or again, ultimately, through no incision at all. Our social responsibility is to prove that new technology improves the patient outcome, and that the price of the improved outcome is *less* than the price of the alternative therapy.

In the next year at Emory University we will be testing a new hypothesis related to outcomes research and cost-effective medicine. One in ten Americans suffers heartburn on a fairly regular basis. About 10 percent of those people are on medications that control acid in the esophagus. The price of these medications is unbelievable—$100 a month, $1,200 a year. Some people take the medications for fifty years—that amounts to $60,000 spent! We can provide effective control of acid in the esophagus with a minimally invasive surgical procedure that costs less than $10,000. The questions are: will it keep these patients off medication? and will it provide them with relief equivalent to or better than the medication? This is outcomes research, and it is another area where minimally invasive surgery may be able to reduce the overall cost of medical care in this country.

Discussion

In response to a question dealing with the costs of procedures, Dr. Hunter noted that most calculations did not consider the positive economic benefit of returning the patient back to work much more quickly. Often noninvasive surgery costs more than alternative procedures; the real savings is in the decreased hospitalization time. Additional savings are realized in the rapid return to work, although this is often difficult to estimate.

In response to a query on optimum technology for minimally invasive surgery, Dr. Hunter noted the importance of tactile sensation and felt that technologies which would allow physicians to work faster—such as a wider, brighter field of vision—and perhaps the use of larger instruments similar to those used in conventional surgery would all be desirable. He said that although there was some debate about the value of 3-D imaging, he personally finds that he feels much less fatigue working in 3-D than working in 2-D. He also suggested that some organizations, perhaps the surgical societies, should get involved in regulating surgical procedures, although at present they are not empowered to do that.

References

1. J.G. Hunter and J.M. Sackier, *Minimally-Invasive Surgery*, (New York: McGraw Hill, 1993).

CHAPTER 20

Minimally Invasive Diagnostics: Imaging

WALTER ROBB
President, Vantage Management, Inc.
Formerly Senior Vice President,
General Electric Medical Systems

"We have to face reality—one industry can't expect to be the golden one forever."

"There will be dedicated body scanners, head scanners, limb scanners, and probably even a breast MR scanner. . . . We will have scanners designed for specific therapies."

"Research will not stop, but industrial R&D support will simply not be sustainable at present levels."

"There is something that is going to help all the modalities—the availability of massive, parallel computers at a reasonable price, which will allow us to increase our computing speeds a thousandfold."

"The next decade will probably be . . . an era for cost reduction and reliability and productivity improvements."

As a participant in the diagnostic-imaging industry for the past twenty years, I share with my colleagues tremendous pride in the industry's accomplishments. The CT and MR revolutions were marked by an unbelievable collaboration between industry, medical schools, research institutes, and academia. During those twenty years there has been continual progress in both imaging performance and cost reduction. In 1978 the CT scanner, a great machine in its day, cost about $800,000; a comparable machine today is less than $350,000. What other segment of health care can show that kind of cost improvement? Today's scanners—with more detectors, bigger and faster computers, and continuous rotation—now cost a million dollars, or about $800,000 in 1978 dollars. When our children are sick, we want them examined on the best CT scanner that is available.

This is an important time for a preview of the future of diagnostic imaging. After twenty years of significant breakthroughs, there is presently nothing on the horizon as big as the discovery of MR and CT. Rather, there are now greatly increased cost pressures and the FDA is moving slower in new device approvals. Although it is distasteful for someone who loves technology as much as I do to face this future, we have to face reality—one industry can't expect to be the golden one forever.

Looking at CT first, it is obvious that decreasing patients' time in the system (or "throughput") and reduction of costs will be the next major thrusts. Technologies such as continuous rotation, helical scanning, and faster reconstruction will increase the output of machines; will reduce retakes because there will be less motion between slices; and will increase the ability of a scanner to screen patients, probably faster than you can get the patients in and out of the room. In addition, auxiliary workstations will be relatively inexpensive, allowing multiple physician viewing without any slowdown in scanning. The productivity of CT scanners will be limited primarily by patient handling time, and that will be helped by having detachable gantrys. The necessity for x-ray tube cooling will continue to be an equipment limitation, even though significant improvements have been made in this area. The next improvements in slices scanned per minute are most likely to come from being able to scan more than one slice at a time. This allows a flat cone of x rays to be used instead of that very thin slice that meant less than 1 percent of the photons produced were being used—the rest being absorbed in the lead around the collimator. Down the road, we will have CT scanners which have a broad cone of x rays that may encompass 128 slices at once. We already have this in industry— looking at the blades in jet engines. This could allow an entire organ to be viewed in one or two passes. This will require massive computers, because the reconstruction job for 128 slices is much more complicated than the reconstruction of only one or two slices at a time; but fast computers will make it possible. At the lower price end, we will see excellent scanners at low prices; hospitals won't need to run extra hours because of scanner limitations. It will be cheaper to buy a second or third scanner than to have the second shift, when a hospital is never very efficient. There will be no reason not to have a dedicated scanner right next to the ER. There also will be some specialty scanners such as those already available which can image the heart in 50 milliseconds and look for calcium in the arterial wall. Special scanners for bone-density measurement will also become available. Even with all this, the CT field will certainly not be as exciting in the near future as it has been in the last twenty years.

In MR, the emphasis will be on customer choice. Every MR scanner doesn't have to accommodate a 300-pound man. Also, there will be choices in accessories, such as multi-element surface coils for showing an entire spinal column. Choices in gradient power will determine whether or not one will have fast scanning capability. There will be dedicated body scanners, head scanners, limb scanners, and probably even a breast MR scanner. In addition, I think we will have scanners designed for specific therapies. Using nonmetal laparoscopes one will see 3-D images *while* working in the abdomen, for example. Hospitals eventually will have as many MR scanners as they have conventional x-ray rooms today.

Unfortunately, the new economic environment will slow research on some of these new items. This is disappointing, because new capabilities are starting to be recognized, including functional imaging, spectroscopy, 3-D blood flow, and heart-wall motion. Research will not stop, but industrial R&D support will simply not be sustainable at present levels.

Conventional x ray is a pretty mature modality—it will soon be 100 years old. However, through electronics, we will have more automation in feedback to set exposures and optimize images, reducing the need for retakes and additional radiation dosage while improving the diagnostic quality of the films. Unfortunately, films and phosphors are about as efficient as they probably are going to get, but eventually the industry will have some form of solid-state image detector that will far exceed the performance of today's image tubes and simultaneously provide high-quality digital images.

Finally, image processing in real time during fluoroscopy will allow a significant reduction in radiation levels. This is important in long therapeutic procedures, not only to the patient but also to the doctor. Cardiologists are limited in the number of procedures they can do today by the amount of radiation they receive. Fast electronic processing will give some renewed excitement to conventional x ray, if only the market can afford to fund the developments.

Nuclear medicine developments will include multihead nuclear cameras and detector systems that capture a greater percentage of the emitting gamma rays, as well as counters that are faster so that even shorter half-life isotopes can be used, making nuclear studies faster, more definitive, and with lower radiation doses to the patient. Progress will come from developments in the biological and chemical areas, such as customized tagged antigens and antibodies. Nothing will match nuclear medicine for its ability to locate multiple metastasis.

Ten years ago, PET and biomagnetism would have received much attention and R&D money, but unfortunately their development will be strongly influenced today by whether the cost per patient can be significantly reduced. That may be more dependent on patient load than on the cost of the equipment. Getting more patients per scanner may mean limiting the hospitals that have those scanners.

In the area of "functional imaging" we may be hurt by having too many contenders, such as MR, PET, SPECT and biomagnetism. It is unlikely that any one modality will obtain optimum support, although a major breakthrough in one of these modalities could change the funding situation. The good news is that government funding is going up. More good news is that there is something that is going to help all the modalities—the availability of massive, parallel computers at a reasonable price, which will allow us to increase our computing speeds a thousandfold. This means that we can now seriously consider reconstructing 3-D images of a patient's abdomen in a reasonable time. We can rotate and slice it, manipulate it, rehearse surgery, and perform simulations at reasonable cost. With advances in fuzzy logic and image understanding, we will be able to segregate specific organs or tissues in an image.

In summary, while there is still a lot of opportunity for improvement in diagnostic imaging, the next decade will probably be characterized as an era for cost reduction, reliability, enhancement, and productivity improvements. It will be very interesting work; however, unless things change, it will not have quite the rate of technical advancement that characterized the last twenty years. Are we smart enough to achieve simultaneously both improvements in performance and lower costs? That may well determine who wins and loses among companies in the next decade.

CHAPTER 21

Minimally Invasive Diagnostics: Biochemical Sensors

ISAO KARUBE
University of Tokyo

"Such biosensors make possible new types of brain research and brain science."

"The fatigue of various individuals can be monitored remotely. We intend to use this system for truck drivers and for airplane pilots."

"In the future, the aged and those who live alone will have an intelligent, sensor-based toilet in their residence—the output of the sensors connected to a telephone line, which in turn will be connected to the local hospital or health maintenance facility."

"These technologies will significantly change health care in the twenty-first century."

My objective is to briefly present the recent trends in biosensor research and development. The biosensor concept initiated in the

United States in 1962 with the work of Clark and Lyons on the measurement of glucose in blood.[1] In 1967 Updike and Hicks[2] produced a glucose biosensor. At about the same time, my group was working on enzyme batteries to develop a biochemical fuel cell using various organic compounds, including glucose, for the battery fuel. We learned that the current obtained from the fuel cell depended upon the concentration of the fuel. We then decided to use such an enzyme fuel cell to determine the components of organic compounds. This was the starting point of our biosensor work more than twenty years ago. We now have been involved in biosensor development for the past twenty years and have developed a wide range of biosensors in Japan, some of which are now commercially available. At the beginning, we were mainly concerned with clinical applications; however, biosensors now are applied for industrial process control, for food analysis, and, more recently, for environmental monitoring and control.

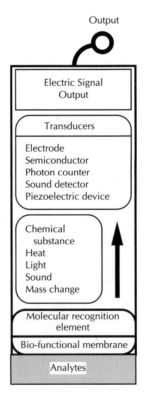

Figure 1. Biosensor Principle.

A biosensor consists of two major components: a biological element, which recognizes a special chemical compound, and a physical element, which converts the chemical-binding event to an electrical or optical signal, which is then processed by a micro computer system. The biological recognition elements are often enzymes. Oxygen or hydrogen peroxide electrodes often constitute the detection element. In recent years, a wide range of semiconductor devices have been used as detection and transduction components of biosensors (Figure 1).

The first commercially available biosensor was developed in the United States by Yellow Springs Instrument Company in Ohio. The first biosensor commercially produced in Japan utilized glucose oxidase, immobilized and fixed on a hydrogen peroxide electrode; it was used for analyzing glucose in blood within about ten seconds. A consortium of twelve companies was involved in the commercialization of this glucose biosensor. Variations on this approach are now being developed for food analysis and for fermentation process control. Enzyme-based biosensors are particularly popular, and various types of enzyme sensors are now commercially available around the world.

Another approach to biosensors is to use living cells, particularly microbes, that are responsive to the special chemicals of interest. *E. coli* microbes, for example, can recognize glutamic acid. They carry glutamate enzymes, resulting in a release of carbon dioxide, which can be monitored with a carbon-dioxide electrode. Such an *E. coli*-based sensor is very robust and can be applied to fermentation process control and for the measurement of glutamic acid concentration in food.

The first microbial-based sensors were used in environmental applications; one was biological oxygen demand (BOD), a marker of wastewater quality or degradation. Classical BOD measurements take about five days, but using a biosensor the measurements can be obtained within about ten minutes. Related sensors are under development for the measurement of cyanide, mercury, sulphur dioxide, nitrate, and ammonium ions—all using immobilized, living cells.

The rapid developments in semiconductor technologies and microfabrication greatly expanded biosensor development. Of particular importance is the ion-sensitive, field-effect transistor, coupled with immobilized enzymes or cells. The enzyme reaction or cellular response leads to a local pH change, which then results in a change in the FET gate potential, resulting in a change in the transistor current, and thus a signal. Semiconductors are easily mass produced. The price of the biosensors can be significantly reduced using such microchip technologies.

Multichannel microelectrodes based on silicon technologies can now be produced, each containing its own different immobilized enzyme. Photolithographic methods readily allow the fabrication of multichannel microbiosensors. We have systems in which seven different systems are immobilized to determine seven different chemical compounds at the same time. The combination of silicon and thin-glass substrate technologies allows for the fabrication of complicated sensors, such as multiple microoxygen electrodes, on one chip. The immobilization of the enzyme or other biochemical recognition element is of course critical. Immobilization technologies are important in maintaining the activity of the enzymes or the cells.

We have worked with ultra-microbiosensors, using carbon fibers as small as two micrometers in diameter. Such fiber-based microbiosensors can be injected directly into tissues. We are now using them with other collaborators in brain research. We can obtain recordings from brain tissue, utilizing a glutamic-acid-sensing microsensor containing glutamate oxidase immobilized on the microcarbon fiber electrode. Such sensors rapidly detect glutamic acid released from neural tissues upon electrical stimulation, thereby directly detecting the neurotransmitter response. We of course are also using acetylcholine sensors. Such biosensors make possible new types of brain research and brain science (Figure 2).

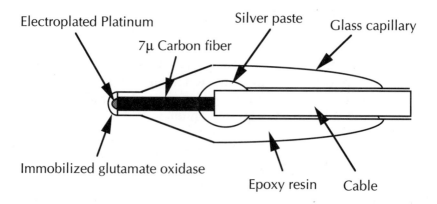

Figure 2. Ultra-micro Glutamate Sensor.

We are now fabricating biosensors on plastic sheets, using various printing technologies. After processing and printing, each sensor simply can be cut off the sheet and used in the determination of various compounds. For example, glucose oxidase immobilized on the sensor becomes a glucose sensor.

A variety of types of transduction systems are available, including surface acoustic wave (SAW) devices, which we are using for the development of flavor- or smell-based sensors (Figure 3). Membranes can be immobilized on the SAW quartz crystal, using Langmuir Blodget transfer technologies. Complicated mixtures of compounds responsible for unique flavors are detected using multichannel chips. Our chips can detect the flavor or smell pattern from various alcoholic beverages as well as various types of food. We are collaborating with police departments, and they are providing substantial assistance to our laboratory.

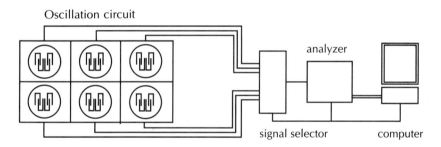

Figure 3. SAW Device Odorant Sensor System.

The detection of odors and smells is important not only to the food industry but also in the medical field. By coupling multichannel biosensor elements onto integrated circuits, the device can provide on-board calculation, signal comparison, and signal analysis. Complete photodiode, integrated-circuit chips are available for less than twenty dollars, permitting the construction of very sensitive sensor systems. We are utilizing this for a freshness sensor. The Japanese like to eat raw fish, and freshness is very important. We are utilizing chemiluminescence with a peroxidase-based sensing system, coupled with this photodiode IC chip, to determine in less than ten seconds the freshness of fish. This also can be applied to pesticide contamination; in this case, we use an immuno-chemical reaction for the detection of pesticides—work supported by the Japanese Ministry of Agriculture.

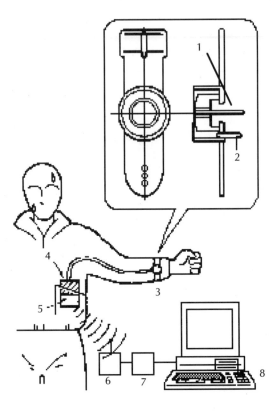

Figure 4. Watch-type Fatigue Sensor.
1—Working electrode (gold), 2—counter electrode (silver), 3—watch-type
sensor, 4—potentiostat, 5—transmitter, 6—receiver, 7—A/D converter,
8—computer

We have recently developed disposable sensors for noninvasive
diagnostics utilizing perspiration and urine samples. Fatigue sensors also are of particular interest, utilizing lactic acid or ammonia
markers. They are designed and built using a watch-type structure
incorporating a miniature FM transmitter. We know that after hard
exercise there is a rapid increase in lactic acid in sweat, which can
be monitored. The lactic acid output, and therefore the fatigue of
various individuals, can be monitored remotely (Figure 4). We intend to use this system for truck drivers and for airplane pilots.
Their condition can be monitored remotely and noninvasively using a simple FM receiver.

The Japanese "intelligent toilet" has received considerable
press. Nearly all of the toilets in Japan are produced by only two

companies; they are sponsoring the research of a post-doctoral fellow in my lab to develop various biosensors to be incorporated into toilets. It will be possible to monitor urine electrolytes and even urine protein concentration via the intelligent toilet. I believe that in the future the aged and those who live alone will have an intelligent, sensor-based toilet in their residence. The sensors will be connected to a telephone line, which will in turn be connected to the local hospital or health-maintenance facility. The signals will be regularly monitored by an expert system, and thus the health condition of these people can be monitored regularly. The expert system can alert the physician or health care provider to unusual situations and the patient can then be called or visited as necessary.

Our final dream, however, is to utilize microbiosensors coupled with microrobotics and drug-delivery technologies. We can envision microrobots traveling through the bloodstream, detecting and removing lipids and plaques in the blood vessels, or detecting and then dissecting cancerous tissues or other unwanted biocomponents inside of the body.

I strongly believe that these technologies will significantly change health care in the twenty-first century. The Japanese government has estimated that the biosensor market will grow to about $17 billion within the next five to ten years. Disposable biosensors will expand this market even more.

References

1. L.C. Clark and C. Lyons, *Annals of the New York Academy of Sciences* 102 (1962): 29.

2. S.J. Updike and G.P. Hicks, *Nature* 214 (1967): 986.

CHAPTER 22

Bioprocess Engineering: Opportunities for Improving Quality and Decreasing Costs of Health Care

CHARLES COONEY
Massachusetts Institute of Technology

"Bioprocess engineering can impact the drug development process: it can improve drug discovery, speed up development, improve process and product quality, and improve manufacturing operations."

"There is a very intimate relationship between the definition of the product and the definition of the process."

"Therapeutic substitution is one of the biggest challenges to the industry."

"Health care cost-containment will cap revenues; at the same time there is an increased cost of drug development."

How can bioprocess engineering improve the delivery and quality of health care at a lower cost ? As we look back upon the changes that have taken place in the pharmaceutical and biopharmaceutical industries, we have seen science through molecular biology create tremendous changes in how we manufacture molecules. This change likely will continue, as bioprocess engineering will lead to better-processed products at lower cost. Yet if this is really going to occur, there are a number of things that have to happen.

There are four areas in which bioprocess engineering can impact the drug development process: it can improve drug discovery, speed up development, improve process and product quality, and improve manufacturing operations.

An often-heard opinion in the pharmaceutical industry is that the cost of goods is not a large part of their selling price—therefore changes and improvements in manufacturing technology are not likely to be important to the future of this industry. Two years ago we initiated a program at MIT involving the Biotechnology Process Engineering Center, the Engineering Research Center, and the Sloan School of Management. We chose to look at the competitiveness and productivity of the pharmaceutical industry. As we began to survey the industry to address some of these questions, we found a resounding answer to the question about the importance of manufacturing: it is and will become increasingly important.

The time line from discovery to commercialization of a drug is on average twelve years. There is a need very early in the discovery process for process engineering to make, at almost any cost, enough material to begin preclinical testing. The manufacturing technology used bears little relevance to the cost-effective technologies needed later on: the need is for enough material for preliminary testing. Later on it is necessary to begin the process of development. It is at this point, the second stage, that it is important to begin to put together a cost-effective process; the product is still seven to eight years away from the point of commercialization. It is at this second stage of process development that there exists the maximum opportunity for innovation. Yet at this point one could well be dealing with technologies that are going to be outdated by the time commercial manufacturing begins. For a number of reasons, once you pass the initial stage of process development, begin precommercial manufacturing, and enter clinical trials, the process is almost frozen—and it is still four to five years away from commercialization!

There is a very intimate relationship between the definition of the product and definition of the process. This has an impact on our ability to develop cost-effective processes with innovative technology. Let us try to understand some of the trade-offs encountered at the early development stage. These are illustrated in terms of an equation which describes the driving force in the commercialization of many products:

Gross Profit = (Market Share) (SA) (SP) (CM)

where SA = Specific Activity, SP = Selling Price, and CM = Cost of Manufacturing.

The selling price is determined by market forces, and therefore by the utility of the drug itself. You pay to get rid of a headache or to dissolve a clot; you don't pay for a gram or microgram of material. So, the specific activity is very important as an early determinant in drug discovery. With cost of manufacturing, you pay to manufacture mass, you don't pay to manufacture utility. This equation points up an important trend that has taken place in the pharmaceutical industries—the desirability of looking for molecules with a high specific activity. A very high value for SA means that one doesn't need metric ton quantities but perhaps instead only small quantities. Examples include the regulatory biotherapeutic proteins that are made in relatively modest quantities. One can envision in the future smaller processing plants, the development of molecules with very well defined, very specific, activities, and, because of the small amounts of that molecule, a minimization of side effects.

As we look to the specific activity of new molecules in the discovery and the clinical trial stages, they do tend to be much more highly active per unit weight. This is a bit of a nightmare, because these molecules are difficult to manufacture. They tend to be very potent molecules—thus the need for containment and special processing is very important. Nonetheless, this represents the modern challenge of bioprocess engineering: the need to make very highly active and very specific molecules—often complex in structure— in small amounts, and to do so under economic terms.

Biologics are molecules that tend to be heat labile, subject to contamination, and somewhat variable in their physical and chemical characteristics. With biologics, as opposed to more well defined drugs, there is a close, more intimate relationship between the process and the product. Many of the products that come forward out of discovery programs are: large complex molecules (proteins, peptides, carbohydrates); low molecular weight (optically active) molecules; specific recognition molecules; and molecules with high specific activity.

What does this mean in terms of bioprocess engineering? A recent OTA report on the cost of R&D in the pharmaceutical industry showed a pattern that has begun to emerge since 1980 in IND applications: an increased number of molecules are going through the FDA-CBER (biologics) route rather than the CDER (drug) route. What does this mean? These are the molecules for which approval of the molecule involves simultaneous approval of the process, hence the great impact that bioprocess engineering has on the definition of these products. The process must be defined very early in clinical testing, and therefore the opportunity for process innovation is minimized. In fact, in many cases there is a negative incentive for optimization. This is one of the great challenges that we have to face. The drivers of change in manufacturing technology are:

- product quality,
- regulatory compliance,
- environmental constraints,
- process safety,
- cost of manufacturing,
- competition,
- generic substitution,
- therapeutic substitution, and
- method of drug delivery.

Definitions of product quality are going to put increasingly tight specifications on the nature of the product and the process. Regulatory compliance with FDA, OSHA, and environmental regulations is putting tremendous constraints on the kind of things we can do. Yet, at the same time, we need to innovate and change, and to demonstrate on a continuing basis that this change and innovation is going to work. This dichotomy is very difficult to manage. The cost of manufacturing needs to come down, but not because manufacturing costs per se have been high. Rather, constraints on pricing, together with the increased costs of doing R&D and increased costs of compliance, mean that we have to find additional dollars. Other factors include increased pressures for generic substitutions and what is perhaps the greatest challenge to the pharmaceutical industry—therapeutic substitutions. There are going to be more "me too" drugs that provide therapeutic substitution.

Drugs with fewer side effects also will be developed as a consequence of new technology. The life cycle of existing drugs will be
shorter and the developer's ability to be recompensed to cover the
costs of new R&D will be less. Cost-effective manufacturing is going to have to bear at least some of the brunt of these challenges if
this industry is going to continue to survive.

Consider the manufacture of insulin in recombinant *E. coli:* the
process involves thirty discrete unit operations. One of my research
areas is computer-based process simulation. These simulations permit us to ask questions and to think about biochemical processes,
not as a sequence of unit operations assembled by the incremental
addition of each step but as an integrated process and complete
unit operation. We can do a lot of "what if" scenarios. We are using
process simulation both in business schools as well as engineering
schools to allow individuals with different perspectives to look at
how to improve, optimize, change, and otherwise understand these
complex processes. For example, the simulation/model can help us
answer the questions: what are the opportunities and what are the
barriers for change in the process of insulin manufacture?

The kinds of changes and innovations fall into two categories:
new processing steps and innovative technologies that allow for the
elimination or minimization of the number of expensive purifica-
tion steps. At this point in the process in development, we cannot
go back and make major changes, because we have to freeze the
process years before it is put into practice. Biotech companies must
develop close strategic relationships with universities and vendors
in order to avoid putting in place processes which are likely to be
cost-ineffective later; this has not yet been done very effectively.

Over the last twelve years the biggest barrier to effective research has been the unavailability of good analytical procedures to
characterize the product in the early stages of process development. A change in investment strategy, particularly how companies do their analytical work, will have a major impact on their
ability to design better processes and on their ability to document
the impact of process change later. Speed to market is key; one can't
afford to do process innovation that will lengthen that critical path.

Alternative solutions or processes may be feasible, such as using a genetic-engineering approach to overcome protein folding or
aggregation problems. A requirement for success is that you need
to know where you want to go, and you have to have the means to
measure where you are so that you can know when you arrive at

where you want to go. One needs to apply metrics to processes, inventories, equipment, and quality control. Our experience is that metrics have not been applied in any systematic matter in the biotechnology industry.

There is a mandate for change in this industry. It has been very exciting taking new science and technology and delivering new products to the consumer. But health care cost-containment will cap revenues at the same time that there is an increased cost of drug development due to increased competitiveness, processing constraints, safety and environmental needs, and therapeutic substitutions. We must improve the efficiency of manufacturing processes, make processes more robust, improve their reliability, and reduce manufacturing costs. Bioprocess engineering then will have an important role in the effective delivery of lower-cost pharmaceuticals.

CHAPTER 23

The Future of Bioengineering

GEORGE BUGLIARELLO
Polytechnic University

"What is wanting is the determination to make it happen. Bioengineers need to take a leading role in the architecture of the system, in its implementation, and in pressing for a rethinking of how the medical profession and the other health care professions operate and are integrated."

"Many of the inadequacies in the prevention of disease occur today for lack of political will. Bioengineers should not stand idly by any longer. We need to help generate that political will.... We can and must do more to change the system."

"Biotechnology will be central to bioengineering—indeed to all of engineering—and bioengineering in turn will be ever more relevant to key aspects of molecular biology and genetic engineering."

"The time has come to look at bioengineering not any longer as a specialized effort tucked into a corner of engineering or medicine but as mainstream engineering as well as mainstream health care and as a key factor in the efforts of our species to modify nature for its well-being and for its future."

Introduction

It is certainly most appropriate when we talk about bioengineering to think about the future, because bioengineering is truly a pivotal discipline for the future of our species. First, two quotations. The much-maligned philosopher Epicurus in his letter about happiness warns us against hubris as well as inaction by saying, "Let us remember that the future is neither totally ours, nor totally not ours." The second quotation is from Peter Drucker: "Long-range planning does not deal with future decisions, but with the future of present decisions."

For all practical purposes, bioengineering is a post-World War II phenomenon. Since the end of that war, the growth of bioengineering has been extraordinary. When I started doing research in bioengineering, at the beginning of the sixties, there was only a small group of people involved in the field; and when you went to visit them you did not need to ask where their laboratories were located—they were almost invariably in the basement or, as in my case at Carnegie-Mellon, in the attic. This book is an indication of how much the field has grown—in universities, in hospitals, and in industry. We must recognize that despite this growth, bioengineering is still in its adolescence and, like all adolescents, is not quite sure of itself, or what it is, or what it wants to be; and it is often frightened by the seeming immensity of the challenges ahead.

The field of activity of bioengineering is very large indeed; it ranges from the endeavor that constitutes the greatest part of our work today, health care, to what has come to be called biotechnology—the application in general of engineering knowledge to biology and, a much less traveled path, the application of biology to engineering. There are challenges in each of these areas. We must always keep in mind Peter Drucker's point that the future of each of them will be determined by our decisions *today*.

The Health Care System

Let me start with the health care system in the United States. I want to make three points. The first is that the "system" is in trouble. The second point is that, paradoxically, bioengineering has contributed to this problem, not from intent or because its products are expensive but because its great technical virtuosity has been applied within the context of a system that needs to be reformed, when it should rather have been used as an instrument for reforming the system. Because of the incentives the system has provided,

bioengineers have worked more at the high-cost end of medicine—
the surgical and restorative aspects—than at the preventive area.
Surgical and restorative aspects contribute out of proportion to the
total cost of health care, and, by so doing, they contribute to
unemployment and poverty, which can kill just like a disease. The
situation is aggravated by the system's failure to control greed.
For example, the high concentration of MRIs created by the shame
of self-referrals absorb resources that should better be employed
elsewhere.

My third point is that we must contribute to fixing the problem.
It is clear by now that the problem has been generally resistant to
government solutions. Even if issues such as defensive medicine,
unfair insurance coverage, or poor control of third-party reim-
bursements are a big part of the problem, what is most essential is
to systematize and rationalize the system. And that is what we as
engineers ultimately are all about—the concepts of system, ratio-
nalization, cost-effectiveness, and feedback.

Most of the technical means for changing the health care system
are at hand. The combination of expert systems, management information systems, high-speed networks, new imaging techniques,
and new sensors and PCs in the patient's home make it possible to
think of a rational restructuring of the system—a new architecture
for it. For instance, long-distance networks and local area networks
involving physicians and their patients, besides being able to connect physicians to expert systems and to each other, can radically
transform the nature of an office visit, the nature of a physician's
training, and our ability to keep the physician up to date. They can
also change the location where health care is provided as well as
the role, influence, and knowledge of the patient. This will help us
create critical masses of skills and at the same time have a more
sensitive system.

The performance of X-ray and other equipment in the doctor's
office will be monitored by specialized health care networks. Costs
will also be monitored, and duplication of tests and records reduced. Patients may be able to carry their records implanted on
their bodies. A much higher level of health care assistance will be
possible in third- and fourth-world environments, which will have
access to highly sophisticated, expert medical systems, networks,
and telesurgery. And, of course, automatic translation of languages
will facilitate the creation of a truly global, real-time, health care
network.

The point, to reiterate, is that almost all of this is technically possible today. But what is wanting is the determination to make it happen. Bioengineers need to take a leading role in devising the architecture of the system, in implementing it, and in pressing for a rethinking of how the medical profession and the other health care professions operate and are integrated.

There are at least three major challenges for bioengineers if we are to take that leadership role. The first is to insist that medical education go beyond the current paradigm. Medicine has become highly technological. The time has come to couple the concept of the physician-scientist to that of the physician-engineer—in other words, a physician who fully uses science but also fully espouses technological concepts such as system, feedback, and cost-effectiveness, and does so not only in the context of research but also (and above all) in the context of medical practice.

The second challenge is to champion the restructuring of the health care system. This is by far the most difficult task for two reasons. In the first place, bioengineers, like all engineers, are reluctant to challenge the system within which they operate. The second reason why the task is difficult is because it not only involves the solution of medical and engineering problems but also, as Keller has so effectively stressed (Chapter 2), a keen sense of sociotechnological approaches—of how technology can change a social system and how a social system is shaped by the technology it uses. Restructuring the system involves many aspects: from empowering the patient, to the creation of physician-patient telecommunication networks, to a wider application of cost-effectiveness concepts, to the seemingly trivial concept of "just-in-time" systems. These aspects of a restructured system are all interconnected. Thus, empowering patients and enabling them to make intelligent choices are matters both of paradigm and of technology—the latter involving, for instance, patient expert systems as well as telenetworks, enabling the physician to be in contact with the patient at home and to be able to intervene, if necessary. This would help decrease the time wasted by millions of patients waiting on the convenience of the physician or the hospital.

The third challenge for bioengineers is to champion new careers in the health care field. We need a new group of health care professionals combining engineering and medical knowledge. To reiterate, we need to infuse the medical profession with the strong knowledge of engineering necessary to reform the system. And we need to develop new careers in the management of health care communication networks—the networks that will enable health care specialists from virtually all over the world to be brought to bear on the needs of the individual patient.

We must do more to change the system. If bioengineers join forces with visionaries in medicine, medicine will become more accessible, more cost-effective, and more predictive and preventive. Sixty percent of all deaths in the U.S. are premature. The fact is that many of the inadequacies in the prevention of disease occur today for lack of political will. Bioengineers should not stand idly by any longer; we need to help generate that political will.

Biotechnology

Let me move very rapidly to the other major arenas for bioengineering, starting with biotechnology. Here, too, I would like to make three points. The first is that biotechnology is indeed a technology—it is a modification of nature. To paraphrase Saddam Hussein, it is the mother of all technologies.

The second point, if one accepts the first, is that biotechnology can be seen historically as a failure of bioengineering, because it is one of the most fundamental modifications of nature that one can think of. Engineering is about the modification of nature; but to my knowledge there was not a single paper, not a single mention by bioengineers of the potential, the prospects, or the reality of DNA replication before those interventions burst upon the attention of the world through the achievement of the molecular biologists. There is, I believe, a profound lesson in that—namely, that our horizons as bioengineers were too limited at the time. Involved as we were in very difficult and exciting work in many areas of living systems, we missed this most fundamental aspect. We have regained ground, fortunately, as our knowledge of instrumentation and processing techniques has become essential to genetic engineering. But the lesson we should learn is not to lose perspective of what we are doing—to think in the most fundamental way possible, dreaming the biggest dreams.

The third point is that biotechnology basically presents three challenges to bioengineering. One is the challenge of industrialization—the scaling up of bench experiments all the way to production. This, as we know, is an area of great importance for our competitiveness, because other countries, without having made the immense investment in basic research that we have made, may be able to profit industrially by it, just as has happened in the field of electronics.

The second challenge to bioengineers is to apply engineering principles to biotechnology. Genetic engineering, the core discipline of biotechnology, is truly an engineering discipline: it deliberately modifies genetic structures; it designs organisms. Thus far it has developed without any major input from engineers. Yet, for the past 150 years at least, engineers have evolved theories of design and highly sophisticated concepts of risk, safety, and related factors. Furthermore, engineering design skills will make it possible to design an organism by computer—to simulate morphogenesis and forced evolution, if one may use that term. The ability, through computer-generated designs, to accelerate time factors and test new biological designs that have not withstood the crucible of evolution will become ever more important to biotechnology.

The third far-reaching challenge in terms of engineering biotechnology is to optimally blend genetic engineering and artificial organs—using them as options or trade-offs when we work at modifying biological organs and organisms. For instance, it is conceivable that the great challenges of the permanently implanted artificial heart or artificial liver will be solved by an intimate combination of nonliving parts and genetically engineered tissue.

In brief, therefore, there can be little question that biotechnology will be central to bioengineering—indeed, to all of engineering— and that bioengineering in turn will be ever more relevant to key aspects of molecular biology and genetic engineering.

Engineering Applied to Biology

The application of engineering to biology encompasses the study and the modification of organisms, including the extension and enhancement of our natural biological parameters. There are still many areas that have received little attention by mainstream bioengineers. One such area is ergonomics—the interface between the organism and outside artifacts. Consider, for instance, the challenge of the humble wheelchair. There are at this moment, in this country alone, 1.5 million wheelchairs, and the potential need is much larger—about 9 million wheelchairs. Wheelchair technology remains very rudimentary. There is a crying need for advanced bioengineering to develop inexpensive wheelchairs that can make it easier to transfer a patient to a dental chair, a car, or a bed, and also to develop wheelchairs or, better, individual patient-transport devices, that can climb steps. I will not dwell on the need for other patient-assist devices, nor on the economic potential of an industry to produce them. Such an industry will not take off, however, without strong incentives.

Biology Applied to Engineering

The fourth major domain of bioengineering is biology applied to engineering—what has come to be called biomimesis. This is the reverse of engineering applied to biology and is a much less traveled road, one of yet largely unexplored importance to engineering. Whether we think of combinations of biological sensors and microchips, of more effective ways of transforming energy, or of smart materials, we see immense opportunities for engineering to be inspired by the highly sophisticated living-systems designs that have evolved following a process that is totally different from the traditional engineering design process. We see, for example, the possibility, however distant yet, to design active materials that combine strength with sensing, communication, self-repair, and energy transformation abilities, without separating those functions and structures as we do today in engineering design. We also see very different approaches to systems integration—an area of potentially great importance to industries that at this moment are struggling with the problem.

The key point is that the direction from biology to engineering makes us aware of alternative ways of approaching the design and production of artifacts. It should thus become truly central to engineering. Among other benefits, this direction can help us solve the environmental crisis by showing a different model of how things can be built efficiently, from simple materials, and with complete recyclability.

Eventually the two directions, engineering applied to biology and biology applied to engineering, will converge. They will converge in the concept of the biomachine—a living organism intimately interacting with a machine to the point that it will be difficult to separate the two components. This may well be our future, as it is already, in part, our present. There will be in effect a Zen-like merger of the artifact and its maker—a merger that will revolutionize engineering design as well as perhaps the very essence of what we are.

Conclusion

The future of bioengineering will depend on our vision in each one of the four areas I have briefly discussed. Regardless of what the specifics of that vision may be, one thing is clear: bioengineers must become far more conscious of what bioengineering represents and of its potential as it straddles engineering, biology, and medicine. The leaders of AIMBE deserve our thanks for the determination with which they have pressed for a bioengineering input in the planning of the NIH and the NSF. We should, indeed, be prepared to contribute to every major discussion and plan about the future of technology and of our society.

The great promise of bioengineering—in health care, in the creation of new technologies and new industries, and in providing a new vision for our future as living organisms—cannot be realized without a change in the context in which bioengineering operates. To change that context, bioengineering must become far more involved in science policy—just as the telecommunications community is doing today with the telecommunications highway, the space community with the space station, or the national computer industry in terms of its competition with Japan. Ultimately, however, science policy intervention by bioengineers cannot be limited to a subordinate support of the genome project or of other NIH programs. It must project a bold vision of bioengineering in all of its four major aspects. These aspects must come to be viewed as a coherent whole, each important to the success of the other ones.

The time has come to look at bioengineering not any longer as a specialized effort tucked into a corner of engineering or medicine but as mainstream engineering as well as mainstream health care—as a key factor in the efforts of our species to modify nature for its well-being and for its future.

Editor's Reference

1. G. Bugliarello, "Merging the Artifact and Its Maker," *Mechanical Engineering* (September 1989): 46–48.

CHAPTER 24

The Future of Health: The Roles of Medical and Biological Engineers

JOSEPH ANDRADE
University of Utah

"Members of communities have responsibilities. . . . They cannot leave these duties and responsibilities to others."

"Our community in general has simply chosen not to be involved. It is not only we who suffer the consequences of that choice, it also is our society that suffers."

"Engineers ... know how to deal with systems, very complex systems, and they can help develop models and means to define and to address such complex problems."

"In some respects we must all do less, so we have the time to do what we do more compassionately, relevantly, and effectively. We need to teach less, but to teach it better; we need to educate in a more integrated and systems-like manner."

"We all hope and expect that a national health care plan will include legal liability reform and improvement of the federal regulatory structure."

"It is time engineers—and bioengineers in particular—began to lead."

In this book, we have been informed, educated, and enlightened by an array of provocative, informative, and well-written chapters. We have also been urged and encouraged to get more intimately, responsibly, and effectively involved—not only in the debate about health care costs and health plans but in the actual redirection of our own individual efforts and activities in reducing the costs, improving the quality, and significantly increasing access to health care in this country and around the world.

Let us consider six points:

- social responsibility,
- national values and needs,
- economics,
- quality, productivity, and efficiency,
- benefits and risks, and
- education and communication.

Social Responsibility

We are each members of a hierarchy of communities: our families, the institutions in which we work and contribute, our city, county, state, nation, and our lovely green and blue biosphere— the planet Earth. Except possibly at the biosphere level, we are members of each of these communities by choice. We could choose to be in a different state, in a different community, and even in a different family. Members of communities have responsibilities: they must be involved in the process of determining the community's values, its needs, and its governance. They should not leave these duties and responsibilities to others.

Unfortunately, the technical community, and engineering in particular, tends to relegate some of its social responsibilities to other members of the community. Often in one's upper elementary and junior high school years there begins to be a number of bifurcations: you are typified as a people person or as an analytical person; you are a life science person or you are a physical science person. Those splits may continue through high school, into college, and finally into our adult professional careers. The caricature of engineers and scientists is that they are not people people—they shun reporters; they have disdain for politicians; and they tend not to serve on school boards, city councils, or state legislatures.

This book and the conference from which it came have argued that we must *all* be involved. Individuals with engineering and technical backgrounds can and should make significant contributions to a range of social and national problems. Their technical and analytical training and background can provide vital input to practically all socioeconomic issues and controversies, whether it be the role of technology in health care, the environment, and the biosphere, or in regard to weather and natural catastrophes. We must *insist* that these important issues and problems be addressed by our various communities and social systems. We must help generate the political will and the leadership to address these important societal concerns.

Our training and background provide a perspective as well as a set of analytical and critical tools. That perspective is often absent or is incompletely and ineffectively presented in sociological debates and deliberations. It is not because people do not want to listen; it is not because we are ostracized or kept from being involved; it is because our community in general has simply chosen not to be involved. It is not only we who suffer the consequences of that choice, it also is our society that suffers.

Those days are now over. We are seeing the development of a new ethic, a new sense of social responsibility in the scientific and technical communities. The old perception—and excuse—of the "two cultures" is weakening. We can look forward to an increasing level of involvement by the scientific and technical communities in the full spectrum of societal problems, and in particular the nature of health and of health care.

National Values and Needs

Engineers rarely attempt to solve problems that don't exist. They like to have well-defined, well-presented problems. The problem with the health care problem, as Senator Durenberger so forcefully put it, is that the problem has not been adequately defined. The problem is *not* just that we spend 14 percent of our GNP on health care; the problem is *not* just that there are nearly 40 million uninsured; The problem is *not* just that we have over 2,000 individual insurance companies, each with their own forms and bureaucracies—the problem is more than that. Samuel Thier said it very concisely: "What the system should be doing is providing the proper balance of screening, prevention, diagnosis, treatment, and rehabilitation." Senator Durenberger went on to say: "What are the real health needs of the people? Is the medical market system with its dysfunctional manner depriving us of the resources we need to meet those real needs? Do we have to change our values to help solve this problem?" What do we really mean by "health care"? Have we defined health, health care, and health policy properly? They are defined very differently in other countries. These are difficult and not particularly analytical questions, and they are the kinds of questions that engineers don't like to address. Engineers and physical scientists chose their professions because they like well-posed problems; they become very uncomfortable if they must deal with such ill-posed questions and problems. Nevertheless, they are *our* problems and, as socially responsible adults and citizens of our communities, *we* must deal with them.

The state of Oregon has been involved in discussions and planning with respect to the general health and well-being of its population for the last five years or so.[1] After many years of public discussion and debate involving all sectors of the Oregon population, the state evolved the Oregon Health Care Plan, which defined and identified *their values and needs* with respect to health and quality of life. The plan addressed the issues of access, quality, costs, and economic constraints, and it formulated a standard benefits package for health and health care, with a major emphasis on prevention, healthful living styles, and early diagnosis. There was a deemphasis on expensive, heroic, and halfway technologies and procedures. The Oregon Plan, and the dialogue leading to it, has generated a considerable amount of criticism, discussion, and debate. It nevertheless serves as a model for what we as a nation and what we in other states and regional communities can do.

Scientists and engineers know that problems need to be at least partially defined before they can be effectively addressed and eventually solved. We really do need to decide if health care is a right, and/or how much health care is a right, and how much are we willing to spend on health care? What do we do about individuals who insist on living unhealthy life-styles? Do we wish to maintain the choice and independence so characteristic of the present system? Susan Bartlett Foote said it very concisely: "Choice has a cost"—and generally a significant cost. Do we want to empower patients to have a significant financial stake and intellectual stake in their health and well-being and in the selection of treatments or nontreatments of their health-related problems? These primarily are all values questions—societal questions that need to be addressed in appropriate forums in order that the problem can be defined.

Economics

What are the costs of health care? Dr. Thier argued that perhaps we need a new calculus, to consider *all* of the costs and *all* of the benefits related to health and well-being. The costs of *your* health and well-being began at the moment of your conception, and they escalated from there. The cost of prenatal care can be allocated both to the mother as well as to the fetus, as can the costs of birth itself. Can we develop a calculus for the total costs and benefits of a human life? If my average life span is seventy years, what will it cost my parents, me, and my community from my conception to my death and burial? We have rarely, if ever, looked at the problem in such an inclusive manner.

Missing a vaccination early in life can lead to significant problems and inordinate costs later in life. We can't simply focus on the incremental cost of that vaccination, or on the incremental cost of the health-problem episodes resulting from a lack of the vaccination. They are all related. The integral stretches from conception to burial. It is an integral which includes an enormous amount of virtually unpredictable statistics and probabilities. Some of us know how to do integrals. Some of us know how to deal with noisy data. Some of us know how to trade quantity in data for quality in application. We can help address those complex problems.

Is the cost of hand-gun control, or gun control in general, a health care cost? Are the costs of drug prevention programs health care costs? And the costs of drug treatment programs—are they health care costs? Is the cost of a summer job for an inner-city teenager, who is likely to acquire both guns and drugs, a health care cost? And what are the health care costs to society at large if that gun-toting, drug-selling, unemployed teenager sells and distributes those drugs and uses that gun? These are all parts of the calculus—parts of this incredibly complex integral. We must now integrate, and not only over the life of an individual and over all of the individuals in society; we must also integrate and consider all of the cross-terms as well. The integral must include all of society. Engineers, at least certain kinds of them, know how to deal with systems, very complex systems, and they can help develop models and means to define and to address such complex problems.

We all know from personal experience that the scientific and technical communities and the medical communities respond to economic incentives. Incentives do indeed matter, and it is today's incentives which drive tomorrow's outcomes. If we can simply identify and define what we want tomorrow, we can implement incentives today which should help drive that outcome. That is again why it is so important to define the problem, so that we can put in place programs and incentives with which to address and to solve it.

Quality, Productivity, and Efficiency

We have seen that quality in the health care system can be significantly enhanced and improved. Improvement in quality and overall enhancement in productivity and efficiency also will lead to lower costs. Productivity and efficiency enhancement does not just mean minimizing labor costs. In fact, it may mean just the opposite. It may well mean taking a little more time to get an appropriate medical history, taking a little time to make the patient aware of his/her medical problem and to educate the patient about the trade-offs of different possible treatments or no treatment as well as to involve the patient in self-diagnosis and self-monitoring. These actions will increase labor costs in the time spent by physician, nurse, or health care provider. But such "increases" in labor costs might indeed be excellent investments in enhanced quality, productivity, and efficiency in the sense of achieving better health and a better health outcome over the longer term. Patients certainly do not want to talk to machines, and they do not want to talk to health care providers who function like machines. They want to talk to informed, involved, compassionate people who can listen as well as pronounce and prescribe.

Hunter and Foote both addressed the issue that there are far too many specialists in this nation, and that the ratio of specialists to primary-care providers is completely out of balance. Incentives are evolving to change that, but they could evolve more rapidly. The same situation is perhaps true in biomedical engineering. There is far more interest in graduate projects that tend to push the scientific and technology envelope, driven of course by incentives from the funding agencies, than there is on projects which may help to solve and meet a current health care need but that may involve more pedestrian or less exciting technologies.

Benefits and Risks

The scientific and technical community tends to have some appreciation of probability and statistics. Those with even the weakest introduction to the life sciences know that organisms eventually die, and that they die from myriad causes. Most of us know that the Gaussian distribution, or normal, curve is more or less endemic throughout biology. Yet, although these principles tend to be part of the education of some college and university students, they are not a part of the education of the general public nor of their lawyers. Unfortunately, these concepts are also not well known among many physicians and medical providers. When they are, they often are not transmitted effectively to their patients.

Keller (Chapter 2) discussed the issue of benefit and risk. Clearly there are more safe as well as less safe activities and procedures. Clearly there is malpractice. Clearly there are poorly designed and manufactured devices; and clearly we need effective regulation with respect to safety and efficacy. But just as clearly there are statistics and there are probabilities. It is no one's fault if an earthquake levels your town or your home. It may be *your* fault for choosing a home on an earthquake fault, if that fact was indeed known to you. Is it really society's fault if you live on a 500-year floodplain? Is it someone's fault if one out of 10,000 medical implants leads to a negative or even catastrophic outcome? Is it fair or right to insist that that device have a one in 1,000,000 failure rate, increasing its development, testing, and manufacturing costs by orders of magnitude to produce such reliability? Is it fair to make the other 999,999 individuals who receive that implant pay the exceptionally high cost required for that level of safety?

Lawmakers and lawyers must come to understand statistics and probability. You and I and our colleagues must educate them. We must see to it that these concepts are incorporated in all professional courses of study—in all majors, on all campuses, in all schools.

Education and Communication

Health care and the costs of health care are important to every single individual in society. We are all involved and we are all part of the problem. Every single group, every component of society, will have to change its own behavior patterns in order to effectively and successfully solve this problem.[2] In some respects, we must all do less, in order that we have the time to do what we do more compassionately, relevantly, and effectively. We must encourage people, ourselves included, to get off of treadmills leading to nowhere, in order that we will have the time to reflect, to identify the problem, and to solve it. All groups must become far better informed and involved in the entire health care area. They must select their physician collaborators more carefully. They must design their experiments—particularly animal and human experiments—far more carefully and efficiently. They must attempt to develop the *societal impact statement*, described by Keller, regarding the future applications and societal impact of new medical procedures or technologies. They must consider and perhaps overcome the technological imperative, also described by Keller, and realize that most ideas and inventions never come to fruition or are never applied, perhaps for good reasons.

Lawyers and judges must be educated—many can be. Letters to the editor, radio and television interviews, discussions with reporters on local cases and controversies—these all help educate the media, the general public, and the law profession.[3] Simple, everyday, elementary-school-level examples of statistics, benefit versus risk, probability, and related topics can have significant impacts, particularly if the entire technical community begins to assume its education and communication responsibilities.

The media often fuels unrealistic expectations; there are many examples of miracle medicines in the media. Health care professionals, biomedical engineers, and others must work with the media to make them more aware of the realities of medicine and health care.

The issue of risks, particularly as applied to health care, must be considered and communicated to the general public and to the media. The difference between voluntary and involuntary risk must be made clear. The role of risk awareness in influencing behavior is critical. The importance of patient choice and empowerment should be emphasized. Cost is unlikely to be brought under control without a general appreciation of the limits of technology and of the inability of devices to correct the natural wear and tear of the aging process. This includes the acceptance by patients of risks commensurate with the statistically demonstrated benefit.

Politicians and elected officials certainly respond to letters and letters to the editor. If they were to receive even a handful of inquiries or statements informing them of risk-benefit-cost issues, they and their staffers would respond. Dr. Healy said, "This puts an obligation on us, each in our own way, to tell the public what we are doing and how it is done. Keep in mind, after all, that the public perception of what we do is not always exact—and when that is so, it is our problem."

Scientists and engineers generally have poor communication skills. Such skills are not fostered in our curricula, and there are not many incentives for developing those skills. There is a general attitude, sort of an arrogant pedestal syndrome, that we don't want to lower ourselves to the level which would be required for dialogue with the general public or the media. Those with communication skills generally do not have the scientific and technical skills, so the information that is getting to the general public, with the exception of that provided by a few good science writers and reporters, is usually incomplete at best and completely erroneous or misrepresented at worst. You and I have to correct that. We have to challenge those reporters, those writers, those lawyers. We have to inform them, and the community influenced by them, that their scientific and technical facts either are correct or incorrect, that their analysis of a technical or semi-technical issue either is appropriate or inappropriate, that their consideration of risk is reasonable or unreasonable given the data and understanding at hand. Not to do so is socially irresponsible—it leads to the system and the problems we have, and the blame becomes ours for being so uninvolved.

Every major report on engineering education, medical education, undergraduate education in general, and public education over the last decade or so has said that we need to teach less, but teach it better, and that we need to educate in a more integrated and systems-like manner. We need to produce graduates and professionals who are good listeners, effective communicators, and responsible citizens. Although I have yet to see a significant response in the higher education sector to these reports, the public education sector is changing rapidly. There are major movements and activities throughout the nation to enhance education at the elementary, junior high, and high school levels, particularly in science and technology education, and that includes mathematics, statistics, and related topics. I am optimistic. As these students move into the college and university environments, as they challenge their professors and fellow students, as they move into the job market and the economy and interact with their co-workers and fellow citizens, I think they will help realize the fulfillment of the hope for a more responsible and involved electorate.

Prognosis and Predictions

Regarding the field of biomedical engineering in particular, George Bugliarello said: "The time has come to look at bioengineering not any longer as a specialized effort tucked into a corner of engineering or medicine but as a mainstream field involved in our efforts to maintain and enhance our species and our planet. But we must first deal with the health care question. That is perhaps the highest immediate priority of the biomedical engineering community." Specifically, we must deal with the following topics and problems.

1. *Health Care and Its Costs.* We must *each* examine the health care, health costs, and health technology fields objectively and decide where our individual talents and interests can be most effectively utilized. Although this book is a significant contribution to such study, it is not enough. There are a number of other excellent sources which should be consulted.[4] More importantly, we must stay current and involved in the ongoing dialogue and analysis of these complex problems.[5] We must encourage our students to learn something about economics, the health care calculus, benefits and risks, and what activities and efforts are needed and could really make an impact.

2. *The Health Care Products Industry.* There is no question that the technological imperative described by Keller and the funding incentives for new technological development have significantly changed. It is therefore unlikely that small incremental improvements in medical devices or technology will prove to be very cost-effective in the new calculus, unless they are accompanied by significant reductions in cost. New inventions and new technologies are likely to be of significant interest only if they represent major leaps or advances in either quality or cost-reduction. Incremental changes will probably be of decreasing interest.

3. *Information.* This volume has made a strong case for enhanced information and communications technologies, and for a computer-based patient medical record that is transportable around the country and even around the world.[6] It is likely that this initiative will

grow and will be implemented. It is also likely that medical-equipment manufacturers will have to design their equipment and their software, not only to comply but to lead in such efforts if they expect to be commercially successful.

4. *More Diagnostic Information.* The availability of rapid, high-speed, transparent information and communication networks, and the ability with them to analyze and cross-correlate large amounts of data from large populations, will drive an interest in having even more information, because the analysis of the information in such large databases will likely lead to new correlations, hypotheses, and insights into disease, treatment, and overall health and well-being. This in turn will drive an interest in even *more* information; so it is likely that there will be an interest in developing large data sets, even for normal patients, as reference and control values. My guess is that early in the twenty-first century when one orders any clinical chemistry, say from a blood or urine sample, hundreds of chemicals will be analyzed at the same time. It will be as easy to do one hundred clinical chemistry determinations on a sample of blood as it is to do one, six, twelve, or eighteen. There will of course be no additional charge for this extra information; it will simply be there because it is expected. Those companies who are used to making large amounts of money on single-test kits are likely to have a very rude awakening when kits and instruments that analyze 50, 100, or even 1,000 chemicals will be available at almost the same price.

5. *Academic Research.* Much academic research in medical institutions is funded by internal funds, often clinical funds "contributed" by academic clinicians. Other academic research is sometimes funded from monies attributed to indirect costs but then utilized internally by the institutions for other purposes. As our national health care plan evolves, it is likely that there will be significant constraints, if not outright elimination, of cost shifting and of the use of clinical incomes for other than clinical purposes. It is also likely that the use of indirect costs for other costs also may be curtailed.

There will be a significant shake-out, particularly in research hospitals and in teaching hospitals' research activities. This will lead to increased pressure on NIH and other funding agencies. The need for health-outcomes research will continue to increase, including the appropriate testing and evaluation of medical devices and cost-benefit-risk studies and analyses. There will be a growing expectation that these studies should be at least in part funded by federal sources. That will make the finite research pie even more difficult to allocate.

6. *Regulation.* We all hope and expect that a national health care plan will include legal liability reform and an improvement of the federal regulatory structure. This will only happen if the scientific, engineering, and medical communities do everything they can to educate the public on such issues as benefits, risks, and costs. If that indeed happens, then there may well be a move to incorporate such concepts in the regulatory structure.

7. *Bio-Based Engineering.* Finally, there is some perceptible motion towards what George Bugliarello called "biomimesis," or what some of us have called bio-based engineering. Bioengineers trained in physiology, cell and tissue engineering, or biotechnology represent Bugliarello's biomimesis, but they are only the tiniest tip of the iceberg.

There is a wealth of biodiversity, much of it going back billions of years and involving millions if not billions of species. Engineers generally ignore it. Back in junior high and high school, you may have either loved to learn to dissect frogs, or you loved to learn about magnets or chemicals. The former sends you on a pathway to the life sciences and perhaps into medicine; the latter sends you on a pathway through the physical sciences and sometimes into engineering. The two pathways rarely meet or intersect in college or university environments or in professional life. Bioengineering and its sister disciplines, biophysics and biochemistry, are exceptions, although even in these cases there is a strong human (or at least mammalian) emphasis. Practically all of the rest of biology is totally ignored. However, the growing interest in bio-based engineering and biomimesis is expected to grow rapidly, leading to totally new solutions to a variety of industrial, environmental, medical, and related problems.

Summary

Senator Durenberger told a little story in a speech in Portland, Oregon, some years ago. He was challenged by an irate constituent as to why he had voted for a particular piece of legislation. His reply: "Madam, sometimes leaders have to lead." It is time engineers—and bioengineers, in particular—began to lead.

Acknowledgments

These topics and opinions have been discussed and formulated over the past several years with many colleagues, co-workers, and other friends. I particularly thank those curious, dynamic, and creative students who have participated in a set of nontraditional courses over the past few years: Critical Science Communications, Bioengineering and the Costs of Health Care, Using Bioengineering for Science Education, and Integrated Science Concepts and Themes. Very special thanks are extended to Dov Jaron and Peter Katona for encouraging the discussion on these important topics.

References

1. See J. Kitzhaber, "A Healthier Approach to Health Care," *Issues in Science and Technology* (Winter 1990–91): 59–65; and H.D. Klevit, A.C. Bates, T. Castanares, E.P. Kirk, P.R. Sipes-Metzler, and R. Wopat, "Prioritization of Health Care Services," *Archives in Internal Medicine* 151 (1991): 912–16; and E.M. Reingold, "Oregon's Value Judgment," *Time* (Nov. 25, 1991): 37.

2. W.L. Lanier and M.A. Warner, "New Frontiers in Anesthesia Research: Assessing the Impact of Practice Patterns on Outcome, Health Care Delivery, and Cost," *Anesthesiology* 78 (1993): 1001–4.

3. J. Marc Adam, "Countering the Growing Skepticism over Medical Technology," *Medical Devices and Diagnostic Industry* (June 1992): 28–34.

4. K.B. Ekelman, ed., *New Medical Devices: Invention, Development, and Use* (Washington, D.C.: National Academy Press, 1988).

S.B. Foote, *Managing the Medical Arms Race: Innovation and Public Policy in the Medical Device Industry* (Berkeley: University of California Press, 1992).

J.D. Bronzino, V.H. Smith, and M.L. Wade, *Medical Technology and Society: An Interdisciplinary Perspective* (Cambridge, MA: MIT Press, 1990).

A.C. Gelijns and E.A. Hahn, eds., *The Changing Economics of Medical Technology* (Washington, D.C.: National Academy Press, 1991).

A.C. Gelijns, ed., *Technology and Health Care in an Era of Limits* (Washington, D.C.: National Academy Press, 1992).

R.S. Dick and E.B. Steen, eds., *The Computer-Based Patient Record: An Essential Technology for Health Care* (Washington, D.C.: National Academy Press, 1991).

D. Feeny, G. Guyatt, P. Tugwell, *Health Care Technology: Effectiveness, Efficiency, and Public Policy* (Halifax, Nova Scotia: Institute for Research on Public Policy, 1986).

V.H. Smith and J.D. Bronzino, "Measuring the Costs of Health Care Technologies," *IEEE-Engineering in Medicine and Biology Magazine* (June 1993): 34–37.

J.D. Andrade, D. Jaron, and P. Katona, "Improved Delivery and Reduced Costs of Health Care Through Engineering," *IEEE-Engineering in Medicine and Biology Magazine* (June 1993): 38–41.

W.L. Lanier and M.A. Warner, "New Frontiers in Anesthesia Research: Assessing the Impact of Practice Patterns on Outcome, Health Care Delivery, and Cost," *Anesthesiology* 78 (1993): 1001–4.

J. Marc Adam, "Countering the Growing Skepticism over Medical Technology," *Medical Devices and Diagnostic Industry* (June 1992): 28–34.

5. An excellent set of sources is the *New York Times, Science, New England Journal of Medicine,* and *Journal of the American Medical Association.*

6. R.S. Dick and E.B. Steen, eds. *The Computer-Based Patient Record: An Essential Technology for Health Care* (Washington, D.C.: National Academy Press, 1991).

List of Contributors

JOSEPH D. ANDRADE, PH.D.
University of Utah

Joseph D. Andrade is Professor of Bioengineering and Materials Science and Engineering at the University of Utah. He serves as Vice President for Public Policy of AIMBE and was Program Chair of the 1993 meeting. His major technical interests and activities deal with proteins at interfaces, biocompatibility, and biosensors. He has edited six books, published over one hundred peer-reviewed papers, been awarded five patents, and served as Dean of Engineering and Chairman of the Department of Bioengineering at the University of Utah.

Andrade's public service and community activities include enhancing elementary school science education and informal science education. He has founded and directs a small biotechnology company, Protein Solutions, Inc., which develops novel materials for science education. He serves as program chair for the Utah Science Center—a discovery-based science center for Utah, to open in 1996. He has a particular interest in targeting and focusing biomedical engineering research and development on activities and developments which can significantly reduce the costs of health care.

J.D. Andrade, Ph.D.
Department of Bioengineering
University of Utah
2480 Merrill Engineering Building
Salt Lake City, UT 84112
Tel: (801) 581–4379
FAX: (801) 585–5361
E-Mail: jdandrad@cc.utah.edu

•

GEORGE BUGLIARELLO, SC.D.
Polytechnic University

George Bugliarello, president of Polytechnic University since 1973, has done extensive work in microcirculation hemodynamics as well as in regional studies of health care. He was president of Sigma Xi—the Research Society; and he also has been a member of the Council of the National Academy of Engineering; a member of the Board on Engineering Education of the National Research Council; past president of the National Association of Science, Technology, and Society; and chairman of the High Technology Council of the New York City Partnership.

In 1992 he chaired the selection committee for the National Medal of Technology. He has also chaired the Committee of Science, Engineering and Public Policy of the AAAS, the Committee on Science and Engineering Education of the NSF, and the Board on Science and Technology for International Development of the National Research Council. He has been a science and technology policy reviewer for several European countries and is a board member of several corporations and foundations. He chairs the Metrotech Committee at Polytechnic University, which oversees the development of Metrotech, the nation's largest urban university-industrial park.

Bugliarello holds an engineering degree from the University of Padua, a doctorate from MIT, and several honorary degrees. He also has been an Alza lecturer. He has published extensively and is cofounder and coeditor of *Technology in Society.*

George Bugliarello
Polytechnic University
Six Metrotech Center
Brooklyn, NY 11201
Tel: (718) 260–3500
FAX: (718) 260–3755

•

CHARLES L. COONEY, PH.D.
Massachusetts Institute of Technology

Dr. Charles Cooney is Professor of Chemical and Biochemical Engineering in the Department of Chemical Engineering, Co-Director of the Program on the Pharmaceutical Industry, and Associate Director of Industrial Activities at the Biotechnology Processing Engineering Center—all at MIT. He obtained his Ph.D. degree in Biochemical Engineering from MIT in 1970. After working briefly at the Squibb Institute for Medical Research, he joined the faculty of MIT as an assistant professor in 1970 and has been a full professor since 1982. He has received the Institute of Biotechnological Studies' 1989 Gold Medal; the Food, Pharmaceutical and Bioengineering Award from the American Institute of Chemical Engineers; and the James VanLanen Distinguished Service Award from the American Chemical Society's Division of Microbial and Biochemical Technology. He was recently elected to the American Institute for Medical and Biological Engineering. He serves as a consultant to and/or director of a number of biotech and pharmaceutical companies and is on the boards of several professional journals.

Charles Cooney's research interests include computer control of biological processes, downstream processing from recovery of biological products, bioreactor design and operation, computer-aided design (CAD) techniques in biochemical flowsheet synthesis, the application of expert systems to enhance process control of bioreactors, the fundamentals of adsorption and filtration in downstream processing, and the use of genetic engineering to solve process problems. A central philosophy underlying research in his laboratory is the use of a multidisciplinary approach in the development of advanced manufacturing technologies for the biochemical process industry.

Charles Cooney
Massachusetts Institute of Technology
Department of Chemical Engineering
Building 66, Room 470
Cambridge, MA 02139
Tel: (617) 253–3108
FAX: (617) 258–6876
E-Mail: ccooney@mitbma.mit.edu

•

C. FORBES DEWEY
Massachusetts Institute of Technology

C. Forbes Dewey, Jr., was born in Pueblo, Colorado, on March 27, 1935. He received a B.E. degree from Yale University in 1956, an M.S. degree from Stanford University in 1957, and a Ph.D. from the California Institute of Technology in 1963. Following five years as Assistant Professor of Aerospace Engineering Sciences at the University of Colorado, he joined the faculty of the Massachusetts Institute of Technology. From 1975 to 1983 he was head of the Fluid Mechanics

Laboratory, and since 1976 he has been a professor of Mechanical Engineering. From 1970 to the present he has been involved in biomedical fluid mechanics, most recently the effects of fluid flow forces on vascular endothelial cells, in collaboration with colleagues at the Harvard Medical School. Approximately 60 of his 120 refereed publications are in the field of biomedical engineering.

He has held appointments as a Consultant in Medicine, Massachusetts General Hospital (1976–80); Visiting Professor of Pathology, Harvard Medical School and Peter Bent Brigham Hospital (1978–79); and Associate in Pathology, Harvard Medical School (1980 to present). In the fall of 1992 he was a visiting professor at the Bagrit Center for Medical and Biological Systems at Imperial College, London, in the laboratory of his coauthor, Professor Kitney. Among other honors, Dr. Dewey is a Founding Fellow of the American Institute for Medical and Biological Engineering.

He is currently a co-director, along with Kitney, of the International Consortium for Medical Imaging Technology (ICMIT), an international organization which includes eighteen members from university research laboratories as well as other industrial and governmental sponsors. Founded in 1992, ICMIT is dedicated to improving the delivery of diagnostic medical images in health care on a worldwide basis.

C. Forbes Dewey
Fluid Mechanics Laboratory, Rm 3–250
Massachusetts Institute of Technology
Cambridge, MA 02139
Tel: (617) 253–2235
FAX: (617) 258–8559
E-Mail: forbes@morgana.mit.edu

•

DAVE DURENBERGER
Senator, State of Minnesota

Dave Durenberger, United States Senator from Minnesota, serves on the Labor and Human Resources, Environment, Public Works, and Finance committees. He was reelected to a third term in 1988 and is very involved in health care policy. He presided over sweeping changes in the Medicare system during the early 1980s. He was vice-chair of the Pepper Commission on Comprehensive Health Care Reform, and is a member of the National Commission on Infant Mortality.

Senator Durenberger has coauthored the Physician Payment Reform Act of 1989, the Catastrophic Care Act of 1988, and the Small Group Insurance Reform Act. He has been very involved in environmental health issues, including such projects as removing lead from gasoline, cleaning up drinking water and groundwater, and the recent Clean Air Act. He is one of the chief authors of the Americans with Disabilities Act. He is an outspoken and vigorous proponent of bipartisan efforts to understand and reform the problems in our health care system. His objectives are universal access to superior quality health care through universal coverage of financial risk.

Senator Dave Durenberger
154 Russel
Washington, DC 20510
Tel: (202) 224–3244
FAX: (202) 224–9931

•

SUSAN BARTLETT FOOTE, J.D.

Susan Bartlett Foote serves as the Senior Health Policy Analyst in the office of Senator Dave Durenberger (R–MN). She oversees health policy issues in the Senate Labor and Human Resources Committee and in the Finance Committee. She came to Washington in 1990 as a Robert Wood Johnson Health Policy Fellow. She has worked with Senator Durenberger on legislation dealing with medical technology policy, reauthorization of NIH and AHCPR, small group insurance reform, health insurance purchasing cooperatives, medical liability, and drug and device regulation.

Susan Foote was formerly Professor of Business Law and Public Policy at the Walter A. Haas School of Business, University of California, Berkeley. At Berkeley, she taught courses in business and public policy and in health law and policy, the latter in conjunction with the School of Public Health. She has a J.D. degree from the University of California, as well as a master's degree in history from Case Western Reserve University.

Foote is the author of *Managing the Medical Arms Race: Public Policy and Medical Device Innovation* (University of California Press, 1992). She has served as an advisor to the Office of Technology Assessment, the Food and Drug Administration, the National Institutes of Health, and the Institute of Medicine. She is presently a member of the Committee on Technological Innovation in Medicine at the IOM.

Susan Bartlett Foote
Senior Health Policy Advisor
United States Senate
Committee on Labor and Human Resources
Washington, DC 20510–6300
Tel: (202) 224–3244
FAX: (202) 224–9931

•

PIERRE M. GALLETTI, M.D., PH.D.
Brown University

Dr. Pierre M. Galletti received his M.D. and Ph.D. degrees from the University of Lausanne in 1951 and 1954, respectively. He is coauthor (with the late G.A. Brecher) of *Heart-Lung Bypass: Principles and Techniques of Extracorporeal Circulation* and has also written more that 200 papers on artificial organs technology, health-care costs, and societal issues related to organ replacement. His academic career in the United States began at Emory University in Atlanta, where he became professor of physiology in 1966. He was named chairman of the Division of Biological and Medical Sciences at Brown University in 1968 and vice-president of biology and medicine in 1972.

He is a past president of the American Society for Artificial Internal Organs (1969–70). He has served as editor of *Cardiology* and currently sits on the editorial board of the *International Journal of Artificial Organs.* Dr. Galletti has chaired many governmental advisory committees, including the NIH Cardiology Advisory Committee, the NIH Data Review Board for the Clinical Evaluation of Ventricular Assist Devices, and the Scientific Project Committee for the Italian National Research Council. He is a member of the boards of trustees of the Morehouse School of Medicine, the Tufts University School of Medicine, and the Institute for Cardiovascular Research of Sion (Switzerland), as well as the scientific advisory committees of several biotechnology companies in the U.S. and Europe. His current scientific interests include biomaterials and bioartificial organs, bioresorbable vascular grafts, piezoelectric polymers, insulin-delivery systems, and the strategy of clinical trials with artificial organs. He currently is president-elect of the American Institute for Medical and Biological Engineering.

Galletti, Pierre M., M.D., Ph.D.
Division of Biology and Medicine
Brown University
Providence, RI 02912

Tel: (401) 863–3262
Fax: (401) 863–1753

•

BERNADINE HEALY, M.D.
Cleveland Clinic Foundation

Bernadine P. Healy was confirmed as Director of the National Institutes of Health (NIH) on March 14, 1991. As director of the NIH, she led a federal agency that has approximately 19,000 employees and has an annual budget of approximately $10.3 billion. In addition to supporting the work of 4,000 scientists located on the NIH campus in Bethesda, Maryland, the agency is the major funder of biomedical research at universities and hospitals nationwide. She resigned as director of the NIH, effective June 30, 1993, returning to her position at the Cleveland Clinic.

Shortly after her appointment, Dr. Healy launched the NIH Women's Health Initiative, a $625-million effort to study the causes, prevention, and cures of diseases that affect women. She also established the Shannon Award, grants designed to foster creative and innovative approaches in biomedical research and keep talented scientists in a competitive system. Under Dr. Healy's leadership, the NIH formulated its first Strategic Plan to guide its research efforts into the twenty-first century.

Prior to her appointment at NIH, Dr. Healy was Chair of the Research Institute of the Cleveland Clinic Foundation, where she directed the research programs of nine departments, including efforts in cardiovascular disease, neurobiology, immunology, cancer, artificial organs, and molecular biology. From the time of her appointment in November 1985, she also served as a staff member on the clinic's Department of Cardiology.

From June 1976 until February 1987, Dr. Healy was Professor of Medicine at the Johns Hopkins University School of Medicine and Hospital, where she also had clinical responsibilities, directed a program in cardiovascular research, and was director of the Coronary Care Unit. In addition to serving on the medical school faculty, Dr. Healy assumed the role of Assistant Dean for Post-Doctoral Programs and Faculty Development.

Dr. Healy has been active in several federal advisory groups. She received a Charles A. Dana Foundation award in 1992 for exceptional leadership in the strategic direction of the NIH, *Glamour* magazine's Woman of the Year Award for her commitment to place women's health as a top national priority, and the Sara Lee Corporation's Frontrunner Award for unprecedented dedication, vision, and commitment to government.

A native of New York City, Bernadine Healy graduated from the Hunter College High School. She received her bachelor's degree, summa cum laude, from Vassar College in 1965 and her M.D., cum laude, from Harvard Medical School in June 1970. She completed postgraduate training in internal medicine and cardiology at the Johns Hopkins School of Medicine. Dr. Healy has written extensively in the areas of cardiovascular research and medicine, and has served on the editorial boards of numerous scientific journals.

Dr. Bernadine Healy
Cleveland Clinic Foundation
9500 Euclid Ave.
1 Clinic Center, S1–134
Cleveland, OH 44195
Tel: (216) 444–0504
FAX: (216) 444–8050

•

SUSAN D. HORN, PH.D.
Intermountain Health Care

Susan D. Horn, Ph.D., is a Senior Scientist at Intermountain Health Care in Salt Lake City, Utah, and an Adjunct Professor in the Department of Health Policy and Management at the Johns Hopkins School of Hygiene and Public Health in Baltimore, Maryland. She is also the Director of the Robert Wood Johnson Foundation Program for Faculty Fellowships in Health Care Finance.

Dr. Horn was a full-time faculty member at the Johns Hopkins University from 1968 to 1991, doing research and biostatistics and health services teaching. She developed the *Severity of Illness Index* with colleagues in 1979 and has collected and studied severity data from many hospitals across the United States. This research became the basis for the Computerized Severity Index for hospital management and payment purposes. She and colleagues also developed an ambulatory patient severity system, and she is developing a nursing acuity measure based on severity data.

Dr. Horn speaks frequently on the topics of severity of illness and quality of care and has authored more than eighty articles and chapters in statistical methods, health services research, severity of illness measurement, and quality of care measurement. She holds a Ph.D. degree in statistics from Stanford University.

Susan Horn, Ph.D.
Intermountain Health Care (IHC)
36 S. State
S.L.C., UT 84111
Tel: (801) 533–8282
FAX: (801) 530–3486

•

ROBERT P. HUEFNER, PH.D.
University of Utah

Robert P. Huefner is the FHP Professor of Political Science and directs the FHP Center for Health Care Studies at the University of Utah. His publications address public budgeting, municipal bonds, the office of the governor, and health policy. A 1992 book, edited with philosopher Peggy Battin, analyzes ethical issues of national health care (University of Utah Press).

Dr. Huefner was on the personal staffs of two Utah governors and a U.S. Treasury Secretary. He was a member of the Commission on the Operation of the U.S. Senate, and has served on numerous state and national health committees. He has a University of Utah civil engineering degree, an M.I.T. master's degree in city planning, and a Harvard Business School doctorate in finance.

Robert Huefner
Department of Political Science
214 OSH
University of Utah
Salt Lake City, UT 84112
Tel: (801) 581–6043
FAX: (801) 585–5489
E-Mail: rhuef@poli-sci.utah.edu

•

JOHN G. HUNTER, M.D.
Emory University School of Medicine

John G. Hunter is Director of the Endosurgical Center, Department of Surgery, Emory University School of Medicine. From 1988 to 1992 he was Medical Director of Laser and Endoscopic Surgery at the University of Utah Medical Center. He is a fellow of the American College of Surgeons (FACS) and a member of the board of the Society of American Gastrointestinal Endoscopic Surgeons.

A renowned expert in laser surgery and endoscopic surgery, Dr. Hunter lectures widely and serves on the editorial boards of: *Laparoscopy and Surgical Endoscopy, Surgical Endoscopy and Interventional Techniques, American Journal of Surgery* (consulting editor), and *Archives of Surgery* (consulting editor). He received his M.D. from the University of Pennsylvania in 1981, and he did his internship and residency at the University of Utah. He is board certified in four states. He now serves as Associate Professor of Surgery at Emory University.

Dr. John Hunter
Department of Surgery
Emory University Hospital
1364 Clifton Road
Atlanta, GA 30332
Tel: (404) 727–8935
FAX: (404) 727–3316

•

DOV JARON, PH. D.
Drexel University

Dov Jaron has served since 1980 as Director of the Biomedical Engineering and Science Institute at Drexel University, where he is a professor of Biomedical Engineering and of Electrical and Computer Engineering. He recently completed a two-year leave to the National Science Foundation, where he was Director of the Division of Biological and Critical Systems in the Engineering Directorate. During his tenure as a division director at NSF, he spearheaded a number of new research initiatives, one of which was "Cost-Effective Health Care Technologies."

From 1973 to 1979 Dr. Jaron was on the faculty of the Electrical Engineering Department at the University of Rhode Island, where he was also Coordinator of the Biomedical Engineering program. From 1971 to 1973 he was Director of the Surgical Research Laboratory at Sinai Hospital of Detroit. Prior to joining Sinai Hospital, he was Senior Research Associate and later Director of the Surgical Research Laboratory at Maimonides Medical Center in New York. His teaching and research have been in biomedical engineering, with a primary focus in the cardiovascular area.

Dr. Jaron received his undergraduate education in Electrical Engineering from the University of Denver. He received his Ph.D. degree in Biomedical Engineering from the University of Pennsylvania in 1967. His major research activities are in the areas of cardiovascular system dynamics and modeling, assessment of cardiovascular function, control and optimization of cardiac-assist devices, and cardiovascular function under stress.

Dr. Jaron is a member of IEEE, the Engineering in Medicine and Biology Society of the IEEE, the Biomedical Engineering Society, the American Society for Artificial Internal Organs, the International Society for Artificial Organs, the ASEE, Tau Beta Pi, Eta Kappa Nu, Sigma Xi, the New York Academy of Sciences, the AAAS, the Aerospace Medical Association, the Cardiovascular Dynamics Society, the Academy of Surgical Research, and the Association for the Advancement of Medical Instrumentation. He is a Fellow of the IEEE, of the Academy of Surgical Research, and of the American Institute for Medical and Biological Engineering.

Dov Jaron, Ph.D.
Department of Biomedical Engineering
Drexel University
32nd and Chestnut Streets
Philadelphia, PA 19104
Tel: (215) 895–2215
FAX: (215) 895–4999

•

MARTHA BRIZENDINE JENKINSON, M.B.A.

Martha B. Jenkinson is a Ph.D. candidate in the Health Care Systems Department of the Wharton School at the University of Pennsylvania. She is the recipient of a Dean's Fellowship, a National Research Services Award, and funding from the GE Foundation. Her focus of study is on health economics and on improving the delivery of medical care. Her current research is in modeling the national health care reform proposals, evaluating the economic efficiency of the incentives, and analyzing their cost-containment implications. She is also working on modeling the dynamics of multispecialty group practice and evaluating outcome measures as they might apply across an entire episode of care, both inpatient and outpatient. Ms. Jenkinson received her M.B.A. from Wharton in 1985.

Martha Brizendine Jenkinson
The Wharton School of the University of Pennsylvania
Health Care Systems Department
204 Colonial 10 Center
3641 Locust Walk

Philadelphia, PA 19104–6218
Tel: (215) 898–6861
FAX: (215) 573–2157

•

ISAO KARUBE, PH.D.
University of Tokyo

Dr. Isao Karube is Professor of Bioelectronics and Biotechnology at the Research Center for Advanced Science and Technology, University of Tokyo. He was on the faculty of the Tokyo Institute of Technology until 1988, at which time he assumed his present position at the University of Tokyo. He holds administrative positions in the International Union of Biochemistry, the Japanese Society for Marine Biotechnology, the Membrane Society of Japan, and the Japanese Protein Engineering and Biotechnology societies.

Isao Karube's major research interests are in biosensors, biochips, marine biotechnology, and environmental biotechnology. He serves on the editorial boards of the following journals: *Biosensors and Bioelectronics; Biocatalysis;* and *Biotechnology.*

Isao Karube
Research Center for Advanced Science and Technology
University of Tokyo
4–6–1, Komaba, Meguro-ku
Tokyo 153 Japan
Tel: 03–3481–4470
FAX: 011–81–3–3481–4581

•

KENNETH H. KELLER, PH.D.
Council on Foreign Relations

Kenneth H. Keller was born in New York in 1934. He attended Columbia University and received undergraduate degrees both in liberal arts (1956) and in chemical engineering (1957). He then entered the U.S. Navy and served for four years under Admiral H.G. Rickover, working on the development of nuclear power plants for naval vessels and land installations.

After earning M.S.E. and Ph.D. degrees at Johns Hopkins, Keller joined the faculty of the University of Minnesota in the Department of Chemical Engineering in 1964 and has remained associated with that department throughout his academic career. His research has included studies of blood-surface interactions in artificial organs, diffusion and reaction in blood flow, fluid mechanical factors in such diseases as atherosclerosis and sickle cell anemia, and mechanisms of mobility. In 1980 he received the AIChE's Food, Pharmaceutical and Bioengineering Division Award for his research.

During the course of his academic career at Minnesota, Dr. Keller chaired the Biomedical Engineering Program (1971–73), served as Associate Dean (1973–74) and Acting Dean (1974–75) of the Graduate School, was head of the Department of Chemical Engineering and Materials Science (1978–80), Vice President for Academic Affairs (1980–84), and President of the university (1984–88). Following a year as visiting fellow and lecturer at Princeton University's Woodrow Wilson School of Public and International Affairs, Dr. Keller joined the Council on Foreign Relations in 1989, where, as the Philip D. Reed Senior Fellow for Science and Technology, he has established a new program aimed at examining the influence of science and technology on U.S. foreign policy formulation.

Dr. Keller has been active in several professional societies, particularly the American Society for Artificial Internal Organs. He has held many positions in ASAIO, including its presidency during 1980–81. He has also served on a number of committees and study sections of the NIH and is a Founding Fellow for the American Institute for Medical and Biological Engineering.

Kenneth Keller, Ph.D.
Fellow for Science and Technology
Council on Foreign Relations
58 East 68th Street
New York, NY 10021
Tel: (212) 734–0400
FAX: (212) 861–1916

•

KERRY E. KILPATRICK, PH.D.
University of North Carolina at Chapel Hill

Dr. Kerry Kilpatrick currently serves as a professor and Chairman of the Department of Health Policy and Administration in the School of Public Health at the University of North Carolina at Chapel Hill, North Carolina. Prior to coming to North Carolina in January 1988, Dr. Kilpatrick was the founding Director of the Center for Health Policy Research and the Director of the Health Systems Research Division,

University of Florida, where he was Professor of Industrial and Systems Engineering, Professor of Medicine, and Professor of Health Services Administration.

Kilpatrick was raised in Michigan and earned a Bachelor of Science (Engineering), a Master of Science (Industrial Administration), and a Doctor of Philosophy (Industrial Engineering) degree from the University of Michigan in Ann Arbor. He also holds a master's degree in Business Administration from Harvard University. His research and publication interests are principally in the application of operations research to problems in health services organization, financing, and delivery. These have included health manpower supply and requirements analyses, optimal staffing for health services facilities, facilities requirements forecasting, decision support systems for multi-hospital systems, computer-assisted clinical decision making, and health care technology assessment studies. He has done extensive policy analyses of the uncompensated-care problem from the perspective of both hospitals and physicians, and he has studied the costs and funding of health professions education.

In 1984–85, as a Robert Wood Johnson Health Policy Fellow, Dr. Kilpatrick served on the health policy staff of U.S. Senator Dave Durenberger (R–MN), who was then the chairman of the Health Subcommittee of the Senate Finance Committee. Kilpatrick was principally responsible for Medicare legislation dealing with payment for outpatient surgery, graduate medical education funding, and preventive health initiatives under Medicare.

Kerry E. Kilpatrick, Ph.D.
University of North Carolina
Campus Box 7400
1101 McGavran-Greenberg Bldg.
Chapel Hill, NC 27599–7400
Tel: (919) 966–7350
FAX: (919) 966–6961
E-Mail: kkilpatrick@sphvax.sph.unc.edu

•

RICHARD I. KITNEY, PH.D.
Imperial College, London

Richard I. Kitney is Professor of Biomedical Systems Engineering at Imperial College, London, and is Director of the Centre for Biological and Medical Systems (CBAMS). Dr. Kitney has worked in bioengineering and health care for the last twenty years; he has published more than 150 papers in the fields of biomedical signal-and-image-processing and the application of computers to health care. He has worked on the study of arterial diseases, cardio-respiratory control, biomedical image processing related to magnetic resonance imaging and ultrasound, and the development of PACS system and 3-D visualization techniques.

Dr. Kitney has worked extensively in the United States, principally at Georgia Institute of Technology, the University of California at San Francisco, and MIT. He is co-director of the joint MIT-Imperial College international consortium on medical imaging technology. He has been a member of both British government and European Commission advisory committees on the application of information technology to health care and he is involved in the formulation of health care policy for the U.K. and the European community.

R.I. Kitney
Director, Centre for Biological and Medical Systems
Imperial College
Sir Leon Bagrit Centre
Exhibition Road
London, SW7 2BT
United Kingdom
Tel: 44–71–225–8509
FAX: 44–71–731–6649

•

DONALD A. B. LINDBERG, M.D.
National Library of Medicine
National Coordination Office for High Performance
Computing and Communications

Donald Lindberg received an A.B. in biology from Amherst College in 1954. After earning an M.D. from Columbia University in 1958, he went on to internships and fellowships at Amherst and at the Columbia-Presbyterian Medical Center. From 1960 to 1968, while a resident, he directed the Diagnostic Microbiology Laboratory at the University of Missouri (UM) Medical Center. From 1966 to 1969 he was associate professor of pathology at the UM School of Medicine. During the 1960s he directed both the Missouri Regional Automated Electro-cardiography System and UM's Medical Center Computer Program. From 1979 to 1984 he was professor of pathology at UM.

The new emphasis on computer technology and data banks led his career in a new direction. In 1969 he was appointed professor and chairman of the Department of Information Sciences in UM's School of Library and Information Sciences. From 1976 to 1980 he also served as director of UM's Health Services Research Center. A pioneer in information and computer activities in medical diagnosis, artificial intelligence, and education, Dr. Lindberg was appointed director of the National Library of Medicine in 1980. Since 1988 he has been adjunct professor of pathology at the University of Maryland School of Medicine. Recently, Dr. Lindberg was named the first director of the National Coordination Office for High Performance Computing and Communications (HPCC). This is a concurrent position with the directorship of the NLM. The National Coordination Office coordinates HPCC programs across federal agencies; acts as a liaison to industry, universities, and Congress; and provides information and communications about HPCC.

Dr. Lindberg has received the Markie Scholarship in Academic Medicine (1964–69), the Surgeon General's Medallion (1989), the AMA's Nathan Davis Award (1989), the Walter C. Alvarez Memorial Award (1988), the Presidential Senior Executive Rank Award (1990), and the Uniformed Services University of the Health Sciences Outstanding Service Medal (1992). He is a council member of the Institute of Medicine and a fellow of the American College of Medical Informatics. Dr. Lindberg sits on the boards of many distinguished societies and associations. He has written four books and authored more than 150 articles, reports, and monograph chapters.

Donald A.B. Lindberg, Ph.D.
Director, National Coordination Office for High Performance
Computing and Communication
Bldg 38A, Rm BIN 30
8600 Rockville Pike
Bethesda, MD 20894
Tel: (301) 402–4100
FAX: (301) 402–4080
E-Mail: NCO@HPCC.GOV

•

C. DOUGLAS MAYNARD, M.D.
Bowman Gray School of Medicine

C. Douglas Maynard, M.D., has wide experience in health care delivery and policy-making at the local, regional, and national levels. A graduate of Wake Forest University and the Bowman Gray School of Medicine, he completed a residency in radiology at the Bowman

Gray/Baptist Hospital Medical Center in Winston-Salem, North Carolina. He has been Professor and Chairman of the Department of Radiology there since 1977. Previously he was Director of the Nuclear Medicine Laboratory, Assistant Dean for Admissions, and Associate Dean for Student Affairs. He is a diplomat of the American Board of Radiology and the American Board of Nuclear Medicine, and he is certified in radiology with special competence in nuclear radiology by the American Board of Radiology.

Maynard serves on the Board of Chancellors of the American College of Radiology (the primary body representing socioeconomic aspects of radiology). He is Vice President of the American Board of Radiology (the accrediting body for all training programs) and a member of its Radiology Residency Review Committee. Past president of both the Society of Nuclear Medicine and the Society of Chairmen of Academic Radiology Departments, he was recently appointed to the board of directors of the Radiological Society of North America (the largest scientific radiology society). He is a member of Leadership Winston-Salem and is on the board of directors of the Winston-Salem Business and Technology Corporation, the Winston-Salem Chamber of Commerce, and Forsyth Technical Community College.

Dr. Maynard is particularly interested in applying classical engineering techniques to medicine. Locally, he directed the development of a prototype image-management system with engineers at AT&T Bell Laboratories. Regionally, he championed the development of a graduate engineering education and research program involving several North Carolina universities, both public and private, with an objective to coordinate the goals of medicine with engineering sciences to improve and reduce the costs of health care.

Dr. Charles Douglas Maynard
Department of Radiology
The Bowman Gray School of Medicine
Winston-Salem, NC 27103
Tel: (919) 716–2466
FAX: (919) 716–2029

•

CLEMENT J. MCDONALD, M.D.
Regenstrief Institute

Dr. Clement J. McDonald has been one of the pioneers in medical informatics, beginning in 1966 as a post-M.D. graduate student in bioengineering and continuing from 1968 to 1970 at the National

Institutes of Health, where he managed the development of one of the
first automated clinical laboratory systems. After completing his internal medicine residency, he continued his medical informatics work at
Indiana University as a faculty member of the Department of Medicine, where he still works today.

His major research focus has been the computer-stored medical record and how it can be used to improve the medical-care process. In
1976 he published results of the first controlled trials of the effect of
computer systems on physician's problems. This large trial of computer reminders included 12,000 patients and 150,000 reminders over a
two-year randomized controlled clinical trial; it showed up to 400 percent improvements in care. McDonald has studied the effects of a variety of computer interventions on physician behavior; for example,
these include the provision of a compact and organized flowsheet of
patient information; display of information about past test results; provision of an empirically based probability estimate that an ordered test
will be positive; and display of test prices when a physician orders that
test.

Dr. McDonald has also been a leader in the development of standards for transmitting electronic clinical data between independent
computer systems. In 1988, ASTM Subcommittee E-31.11, which he
chaired, published the first fully qualified consensus standard for clinical data interchange. He continues to foster the development and use
of standards as chairman of ASTM E-31.11 and HL7's order-entry,
clinical-data-reporting subcommittees, and is chairman of the American National Standards Institute (ANSI) planning panel on medical informatics.

Dr. McDonald has been a leader in professional societies of medical informatics; he was a board member and officer of the Symposium
for Clinical Informatics. He was a founding board member, and is now
president, of the American Medical Informatics Association; he has
been active in national review committees for a variety of agencies,
and is currently a member of the IOM Committee on Guidelines.

Clement McDonald
Indiana University School of Medicine
Regenstrief Institute for Health Care
1001 W. 10th Street
Fifth Floor
Indianapolis, IN 46202
Tel: (317) 630–7070
FAX: (317) 630–6962
E-Mail: clem@regen.rg.iupui.edu

•

MICHAEL NELSON, PH.D.
Office of Science and Technology Policy

Michael Nelson has worked with Vice President Albert Gore for more than five years on science and technology issues, responsible for issues ranging from computer technology to earthquake research to biotechnology. He was the lead Senate staffer on then-Senator Gore's high-performance computing legislation and other related information technology bills.

Nelson has a B.S. in geology from Caltech and a Ph.D. in geophysics from M.I.T. When Albert Gore moved from the Senate to the White House, Nelson followed and is now working at the White House Office of Science and Technology Policy, where he continues to work on a range of issues, including information technology and information policy.

Michael Nelson
Office of Science and Technology Policy (OSTP)
The White House
1600 Pennsylvania Ave, NW
Washington, DC 20500
Tel: (202) 395–6175
FAX: (202) 395–4155
E-Mail: mnelson@ostp.eop.gov

•

ROBERT M. NEREM, PH.D.
Georgia Institute of Technology

Dr. Robert Nerem was appointed in 1987 as the Parker H. Petit Professor, and he became one of six Institute Professors at Georgia Tech in Fall 1991. He received his Ph.D. in 1964 from Ohio State University and joined the faculty there in Aeronautical and Astronautical Engineering, being promoted to professor in 1972. He served from 1975 to 1979 as Associate Dean for Research in the Ohio State University Graduate School. From 1979 to 1986 he was professor and Chairman of the Department of Mechanical Engineering at the University of Houston. At the beginning of 1987 he joined Georgia Tech.

Nerem is the author of more than eighty journal articles. He is President of the International Union for Physical and Engineering Sciences in Medicine and is immediate past president of the International Federation for Medical and Biological Engineering (1988–91). He served as technical editor, *ASME Journal of Biomechanical Engineering*

(1988–92). In 1988 Professor Nerem was elected to the National Academy of Engineering, and in 1992 to the Institute of Medicine of the National Academy of Sciences. His research interests include biofluid mechanics, cardiovascular devices, cellular engineering, vascular biology, atherosclerosis, and tissue engineering. He is founding president of the American Institute for Medical and Biological Engineering.

Nerem, Robert M., Ph.D.
School of Mechanical Engineering
Georgia Institute of Technology
Atlanta, GA 30332-0405
Tel: (404) 894–2768
Fax: (404) 894–2291

•

WILLIAM P. PIERSKALLA, PH.D.
University of California at Los Angeles

William P. Pierskalla is a professor and Dean of the John E. Anderson Graduate School of Management at UCLA. He holds a B.A. in Economics, an M.B.A. degree from Harvard University, an M.A. in Mathematics from the University of Pittsburgh, an M.S. in Statistics, and a Ph.D. in Operations Research from Stanford University. His current research interests include operations research, operations management, issues of global competition, and the management aspects of health care delivery.

Dr. Pierskalla is a past president of the International Federation of Operational Research Societies (1992–94); is on the editorial advisory board of *Production and Operations Management;* is a past president of the Operations Research Society of America; and is past editor of *Operations Research.* He recently was the Deputy Dean for Academic Affairs, the Director of the Huntsman Center for Global Competition and Leadership, and the Chairman of the Health Care Systems Department at the Wharton School of the University of Pennsylvania. He lectures at universities and organizations in the United States, Europe, and Japan and has published more than fifty refereed articles in mathematical programming, transportation, inventory and production control, maintainability, and health care delivery.

William P. Pierskalla, Ph.D.
Dean, Anderson Graduate School of Management
University of California at Los Angeles (UCLA)
Los Angeles, CA 90024

Tel: (310) 825–7982
FAX: (310) 206–2002
E-Mail: wpierska@agsm.ucla.edu

•

WALTER ROBB, PH.D.
President, Vantage Management, Inc.

Walter L. Robb was formerly senior vice president for corporate research and development at General Electric Company and a member of the company's Corporate Executive Council. Dr. Robb started his career with General Electric in 1951 as a chemical engineer at the Knolls Atomic Power Laboratory; he became head of the Medical Systems Division in 1973 and became senior vice president for research and development in 1986. He holds patents related to permeable membranes and separation processes and is widely published. He was vice chairman of the board of regents of the Milwaukee School of Engineering, served on the board of directors of the Health Industry Manufacturers Association, and is a member of the National Academy of Engineering.

Dr. Robb holds a B.S. degree in Chemical Engineering from Pennsylvania State University, and has M.S. and Ph.D. degrees in Chemical Engineering from the University of Illinois. He retired from the General Electric Corporation in 1993 and is now a private consultant.

Walter L. Robb
President, Vantage Management, Inc.
1222 Troy Road
Schenectady, NY 12309
Tel: (518) 782–0050
FAX: (518) 782–0030

•

RICHARD M. SATAVA, M.D., F.A.C.S.
Advanced Research Projects Agency (ARPA)

Richard Satava, M.D., F.A.C.S. is a practicing clinical and research general surgeon in the active duty Army Medical Corps, currently assigned to ARPA. His undergraduate training was at the Johns Hopkins University. He attended medical school at Hahnemann University of Philadelphia, with an internship at the Cleveland Clinic, surgical residency at the Mayo Clinic, and a fellowship with a Master of Surgical

Research degree at Mayo Clinic. He has been active in surgical education and surgical research, and he has over fifty publications and book
chapters in diverse areas of advanced surgical technology, including
surgery in the space environment, video and 3-D imaging, telepresence surgery, and the virtual-reality surgical simulator.

During sixteen years of military surgery, Satava has been an active
flight surgeon, an army astronaut candidate, a MASH surgeon for the
Grenada invasion, and a medical commander during operation Desert
Storm—all while continuing a full-time clinical surgical service. While
striving to practice the complete discipline of surgery, he is aggressively pursuing the leading edge of advanced technologies and applying them to develop the next generation of surgery, what has been
called Surgery: 2001.

Dr. Richard Satava
DIRO/Biomedical Technology
Advanced Research Projects Agency
3701 North Fairfax Drive
Arlington, VA 22203–1714
Tel: (703) 696–2265
FAX: (703) 696–2201
E-Mail: rsatava@arpa.mil

•

SAMUEL O. THIER, M.D.
Brandeis University

Samuel O. Thier is the sixth president of Brandeis University. He
came to Brandeis on September 1, 1991, after serving six years as president of the Institute of Medicine, National Academy of Sciences. Prior
to that he served for eleven years as chairman of the Department of Internal Medicine at Yale University School of Medicine, where he was
also Sterling Professor.

Dr. Thier is a nationally known, widely published authority on internal medicine and kidney disease. He is equally well known for his
expertise in the areas of national health policy, medical education, and
biomedical research.

Born in Brooklyn, New York, on June 23, 1937, he attended Cornell
University and received his medical degree in 1960 from the State University of New York at Syracuse. After medical school he served on the
medical staff of Massachusetts General Hospital, first as an intern and
resident and later as chief resident in medicine and chief of the Renal
Unit; he also served in the U.S. Public Health Service National Insti-

tutes of Health. Prior to joining the faculty at Yale in 1975, he held faculty appointments in the medical schools at Harvard University and the University of Pennsylvania.

Thier holds honorary doctorates from the State University of New York, Tufts University, George Washington University, Rush University, Mount Sinai School of Medicine of the City University of New York, Hahnemann University, the Medical College of Pennsylvania, and Virginia Commonwealth University. He is the recipient of the UCSF Medal of the University of California, San Francisco. He has served as president of the American Federation of Clinical Research and as chairman of the American Board of Internal Medicine. He is a Master of the American College of Physicians and is a Fellow of the American Academy of Arts and Sciences.

Samuel Thier, President
Brandeis University
415 S. Street
Waltham, MA 02254–9110
Tel: (617) 736–3001
FAX: (617) 736–3016

•

BURTON A. WEISBROD, PH.D.
Northwestern University

Burton Weisbrod is John Evans Professor of Economics and Director of Northwestern University's Center for Urban Affairs and Policy Research. He was, until July 1990, Evjue-Bascom Professor of Economics at the University of Wisconsin, where he had been on the faculty since 1964 and where he had founded and directed the Center for Health Economics and Law. He was born in Chicago, receiving his undergraduate degree in Management from the University of Illinois, and his M.A. and Ph.D. degrees in Economics from Northwestern University. Weisbrod has held visiting faculty appointments at Brandeis, Harvard, Princeton, and Yale universities, and abroad at the Australian National University and the University Autonoma de Madrid. In addition, he was a senior staff member of the Council of Economic Advisers to Presidents John F. Kennedy and Lyndon B. Johnson.

Weisbrod's elected positions include: Fellow of the American Association for the Advancement of Science (AAAS), member of the Institute of Medicine of the National Academy of Sciences, member of the Executive Committee of the American Economic Association, and president of the Midwest Economic Association. He is the author or coauthor of nine books, editor of four, and author of more than one hundred articles in professional journals and books.

His research has focused on public policy analysis in the areas of economics of education, health, medical research, manpower, public interest law, the military draft, benefit-cost analysis, and, most recently, philanthropy, voluntarism, and the nonprofit sector. Consulting widely for governments, foundations, nonprofit organizations, and private firms in the United States, Europe, and Asia, Weisbrod has also served on numerous national and international study and conference committees and has been on the editorial boards of six journals.

Dr. Burton Weisbrod
Center for Urban Affairs and Policy Research
Northwestern University
Evanston, IL 60208
Tel: (708) 491–3395
FAX: (708) 491–9916

•

JOHN E. WENNBERG, M.D.
Dartmouth Medical School

John E. Wennberg, M.D., M.P.H., is the Director of the Center for the Evaluative Clinical Sciences and Professor of Epidemiology at Dartmouth Medical School. He is a nationally recognized leader in efforts to reform the doctor-patient relationship and improve the delivery of quality health care to all Americans. His wide-ranging public presentations to medical gatherings, public interest groups, and congressional hearings, as well as his commentaries on editorial pages and in the electronic media, have gained attention around the nation. Dr. Wennberg currently serves on the Institute of Medicine's Health Sciences Policy Board and on the Committee on Technological Innovation in Medicine. As a founder and continuing board member of the Foundation for Medical Decision Making, he was instrumental in the design of interactive videodiscs for use by patients to help them share with their physicians in the decision-making process about treatment.

Dr. Wennberg began his academic research with work regarding why similar geographical areas may present dramatically different rates for certain surgical procedures. Building on this research, his professional writings now explore outcomes research, patient preferences, the changing role of primary-care physicians, and the effect of the supply of resources on the patterns of utilization. Wennberg is also the principal investigator for the Prostate Assessment Team, established under a new federal government program for outcomes research. He is a graduate of Stanford University and the McGill Medical School in Montreal.

John E. Wennberg, M.D.
Director, Center for the Evaluative Clinical Sciences
Dartmouth Medical School
7250 Strasenburgh
Hanover, NH 03755–3863
Mary Cloud (603) 650–1684
FAX: (603) 650–1225
E-Mail: j.wennberg@dartmouth.edu

•

GAIL WILENSKY
Project Hope

Gail Wilensky is currently a senior fellow at Project Hope, an international health foundation, where she was a vice president for health affairs from 1983 to 1990. She was the health and welfare advisor to President George Bush and before that directed the Health Care Financing Administration (HCFA), the agency that runs the Medicare and Medicaid Program. She is a health economist by training and has done extensive research in the problems of the uninsured and the costs of health care. She has written and spoken on these topics frequently and is a member of the Institute of Medicine.

Gail Wilensky
Project Hope
Carter Hall
Millwood, VA 22646
Tel: (301) 656–7401 x 260
FAX: (301) 654–0629 or 0621

Index

Jenkinson, Martha B., 43, 217
Johnson, Samuel, 121
Judges, 199
"Just-in-time" systems, 187

Karube, Isao, 171, 218
Keller, Kenneth H., 12, 36, 187, 198, 218
Kickbacks, 162
Kilpatrick, Kerry, 57, 219
Kitney, Richard I., 127, 220
Kitzhaber, J., 204
Krebs cycle, 63
Krebs, Hans, 63

Lactic acid, 176
Languages, 186
Laparoscopic cholecystectomy, 161
Laparoscopic surgery, 93, 96, 160
Lawyers, viii, 115, 198
Leadership, 187
Least squares, 123
Liability, 12, 32
    reform of, 192, 203
Libraries, 105
Library of Congress, 105
Lifelong learning, 105, 113
Limb scanners, 168
Lindberg, Donald A.B., 113, 221
Link, Edwin, 95
Lipmann, Fritz, 63
Lithotripter, 9
Liver transplant, 80
Loansome Doc, 115
Los Angeles, 28

Magnetic resonance imaging (MRI), 130
Maine, 151
Malpractice, 124, 198
Mammography, 7, 121
Managed care, 48
Managed competition, 37, 38, 47
Manufacturing, 105, 179
Massachusetts, 150, 178
Massachusetts Institute of Technology,
    208, 209
Maynard, Douglas D., 144, 222
Mayo Clinic, 27, 50, 103
McDonald, Clement J., 102, 118, 223
Media, 199
Medical education, 113, 187, 200
Medical engineers, 192
Medical equipment, 127
Medical imaging, 127, 130
Medical informatics, 93, 117
Medical market system, 27
Medical practice, 122, 187
Medical records, 103, 105, 107, 118, 123,
    124

Medical schools, 40, 87
Medical technology, 4, 5, 20, 89
MEDINET, 134
MEDLARS, 114
MEDLINE, 114
Menopausal bleeding, 150
Metastasis, 169
Microsurgery, 97
Middle class, 31, 43
Military Medical System, 93
Minimally invasive surgery, 93, 157
Minneapolis—St. Paul, 28
Minnesota, 28, 46, 50, 210
Miracle medicines, 199
Molecular biology, 184
Monitoring, integrated, 90
MR, 169
Multimedia, 138
Myocardial infarction, 156

NASA, 104
National Academy of Sciences, x
National Health Board, 48
National information infrastructure, 119
National Institute of Standards and
    Technology (NIST), 107
National Institutes of Health, 60
National Library of Medicine, 113, 221
National Research and Education
    Research (NRER), 116
National Science Foundation (NSF), x, 88
Nelson, Michael, 101, 225
Nerem, Robert M., 225
Nerve regeneration, 10
Network, 102, 140, 145
Neurology, 130
Neurotransmitter, 174
New York, 184
NIH Strategic Plan, 62
Nintendo, 94
Nonlinear regression, 123
North Carolina, 58
Northwestern University, 229
Nuclear medicine, 169
Nurse, 197
Nutrition, 10, 69

Obstetrics, 130
Odor sensors, 175
Office of Science and Technology Policy,
    225
Oncology, 130
Open architecture, 137
Open-loop systems, 128
Operation research, 57, 90
Oregon, 84, 195, 203
Oregon Plan, 19, 24
Organ transplantation, 80